BOYFRIEND
11

A Gay Guy's Guide to Dating,
Romance, and Finding True Love

JIM SULLIVAN

(V)

VILLARD / NEW YORK

2003 Villard Books Trade Paper Original

Copyright © 2003 by Jim Sullivan

All rights reserved under International and Pan-American Copyright
Conventions. Published in the United States by Villard Books, an imprint of
The Random House Ballantine Publishing Group, a division of
Random House, Inc., New York, and simultaneously in Canada
by Random House of Canada Limited, Toronto.

VILLARD and "V" CIRCLED Design are registered trademarks
of Random House, Inc.

Library of Congress Cataloging-in-Publication Data

Sullivan, Jim.
Boyfriend 101 : a gay guy's guide to dating, romance, and
finding true love / Jim Sullivan.
p.   cm.
ISBN 0-8129-9219-9
1. Gay men—Social life and customs. 2. Gay men—Psychology. 3. Dating (Social
customs) 4. Mate selection. I. Title: Boyfriend one hundred one. II. Title:
Boyfriend one hundred and one. III. Title.
HQ76 .S83 2003
305.38'9664—dc21   2002191045

Villard Books website address: www.villard.com

Printed in the United States of America

24689753

Book design by Casey Hampton

BOYFRIEND 101

TO MY PARENTS,

John F. Sullivan & Florence Sullivan

TO MY GAY BROTHERS AND LESBIAN SISTERS,

those living and those passed on

ACKNOWLEDGMENTS

To my wonderful editor, Tim Farrell, whose generosity of spirit and patience helped me see the total picture. To Bruce Tracy and everyone at Random House and Villard.

To all the fabulous gay men I have worked with over the years. You were the inspiration for this book.

To Ram Dass, who helps me "be here now." To Mary Cropper, CSW, who encouraged me from the start.

To Malaga Baldi; Ellen Roberts; Katherine Crowley; Bob Morris; Blandon Belushin; Jack Schelgel and Out Professionals. To Cynthia O'Neal, Eric Schneider, and everyone at Friends in Deed. To Norbert Sinski; Michael Gast, CSW; Dr. Michael Schroeder; Stephen McFadden, CSW; Walter Zeichner; Susan Lee; David Jackson; Karl Stewart; Patrick Hennessey, M.D.; Marble Collegiate Church; Congregation Beth Simchat Torah; Jim Varriale; Barry Malvin; David Harvey Studios; Joe Windish, Robert Woodworth, and LGBT Center, New York City; David

Flower in Provincetown; Bruce Eberhardt; Richard Marfuggi, M.D.; David Colbert, M.D.; Martin Algaze; Gay Men's Health Crisis; Fenway Community Health Center. To Kripalu, which provides me a home away from home. To Esalen, which is just one step from heaven. To Bill W. and Lois.

To all my fellow steppers at Malibu and my very special men's meeting.

To the School Sisters of St. Francis (Milwaukee), who gave me love and taught me how to diagram a sentence.

To *all* my support angels and friends (you know who you are), including Peter Eurich, Rose Meehan, John Carrigan, Reed Kelly, Lou Martarano, Ken Cottrell, Don Leight, Arnie Kolodner, and Bill Shattls, who blesses me from beyond.

To my brothers and sisters: Dennis, John, Kathryn, Rita, and Joseph Kevin, who left us much too soon.

CONTENTS

INTRODUCTION

As you begin reading *Boyfriend 101,* you will encounter the stories of men in whose experiences you may see yourself mirrored. It should be a relief for you to discover you're not alone in finding dating a sometimes difficult endeavor. You may also discover there is no such thing as the perfect date or the perfect relationship. Dating is a process that often leads to a highly desirable result—a long-term, loving relationship. But dating is more than a means to an end. It can be an end in itself. It's a process that I ask you—and you should ask yourself—to be open to.

LAWRENCE, THIRTY-ONE

Lawrence, a thirty-one-year-old graphic designer, came to me for a consultation because he felt his dating life was "in the pits." He went on several dates a month, but they never seemed to amount to anything more than a friendly dinner or, occasionally, a prelude to sex. Some guys he really liked would not return phone calls after the first date; or he wouldn't return the calls of others who really liked him, if he felt they didn't "click." Lawrence feared he was just part of "The Big Chase": men running after one another, but not really connecting in any meaningful way.

Lawrence's past relationships included a semester-long romance his senior year of college and a five-month involvement with a guy he met at his gym. His other "relationships" were really serial flings, each lasting no longer than a month. Not having a long-term relationship made Lawrence ashamed, since he felt that all of his friends and acquaintances were happily coupled. He believed he had to meet someone by the time he reached thirty—and had sworn to himself that he would—because he felt certain the pool of attractive, available men would diminish as he grew older.

I told Lawrence there's no shame in not having met a man by age thirty-*one*. In my work as a relationship counselor in the gay community, I have witnessed men meet life partners at thirty, forty, and fifty years of age, and beyond. Age—which is just a number in the head—can cause needless panic unless we're gentle with ourselves and accept wherever we're at along the dating spectrum. Finding a mate is not a race. Some men even choose to remain single, happily.

Lawrence primarily met eligible men at bars/clubs or through online gay dating services. It wasn't hard for Lawrence to meet guys in bars, particularly after a few drinks, but getting a little drunk almost always led to bringing someone home for sex and often never seeing him again. And meeting singles online was not as successful as he thought it might be. He posted a sexy photo of himself—wearing Levi's but no shirt—which mostly attracted guys who only wanted sex. Lawrence felt flattered by these sexually charged responses, but the experience amounted to nothing more than virtual cruising.

He got a new photo—this time, with a shirt—and although he attracted fewer men, the responses were more serious. Among the ten or so guys he met through the dating service, two were really top-notch, but—when they met for coffee—didn't turn him on sexually. Lawrence was confused. How can guys be attractive in so many ways, but not sexually? I had to tell him it can sometimes take more than a few dates to feel sexual attraction. Besides, I suggested, in the future he should not close himself off to the possibility of meeting men who might become friends.

Like Lawrence, men new to the dating scene—or returning to dating after a long-term relationship ends—can benefit from creating a dating action plan. A coherent, well-organized plan of action provides structure for what can otherwise be an overwhelming experience. Again, dating is a process. Husbands don't land at your door just because you wish it would happen! As part of the dating strategy Lawrence and I created, he planned to:

- expand his network of gay friends, thereby providing a firm emotional foundation for his personal life
- determine precisely what he wanted and needed in another man
- join two gay organizations (social, sports, religious) over a one-month period, and attend at least three organizational events

- rewrite his online profile and also write a personal ad for his local gay newspaper
- make two to four dates a month
- keep to this simple guideline: no sex for the first three dates

The easiest part of Lawrence's dating plan was joining two gay organizations: he chose a local gay political group and became a member of the Gay Men's Chorus. Within two months, he had begun cultivating several new friendships and was linked to a larger network of gay men.

Previously, Lawrence had not really thought about what he wanted and needed in another man. As long as a guy was smart, good-looking, and had a job, Lawrence thought he was a good catch. Qualities like honesty, emotional support, commitment, and stability did not appear on Lawrence's dating radar screen. When I asked Lawrence to make a list of what he wanted in another man, he was a bit shocked to realize he had let these factors slip by him in the past.

Lawrence went on three dates within six weeks of our first consultation. "No sex for the first three dates" was the most difficult challenge for him, as it is for most gay men. Concentrating on getting to know someone, and opening oneself up to another man, is, undeniably, tough work: after the first couple of dates, Lawrence's impulse was either to call it quits or to have sex with the guy and then end it. But really dating—consciously—means growing up and making informed choices about who we want in our lives as friends, family, and lovers. It takes time, commitment, and perseverance to get the love we want in our lives.

Lawrence met Andrew, a thirty-six-year-old journalist, at a political fund-raiser, and was captivated by his boyish good looks and engaging personality. They exchanged numbers and, the next day, arranged to meet for dinner. The evening went off without a hitch, except at the end, when Andrew invited Lawrence back to his place and Lawrence said he didn't want to go home with Andrew since he didn't want to start "fooling around" on the first date. Andrew insisted that they didn't have to "fool around"—he just wanted to have Lawrence over for coffee. Lawrence agreed, but got more than the coffee he'd bargained for. As soon as Andrew shut his apartment door, they started kissing. In ten minutes, they were in bed having what was, for Lawrence, intense sex. The next day, Lawrence called Andrew and left a message on his machine saying what a wonderful time he had had. No return call. Lawrence called Andrew three times over the next week and still got no response. Finally, Andrew e-mailed him: "Lawrence—Sorry for not getting back. Been overwhelmed with work. Will be in Japan on business for a week and will call you when I get back. Andrew." But Andrew never called.

Lawrence couldn't understand. "I definitely got mixed signals. During sex, Andrew told me, 'You're so handsome. I could easily fall in love with you. I'm not going to let you slip by!' Why would he say that and not return my calls?" He asked me if he should call Andrew again.

I said no. Lawrence's best bet was to move on and date other guys. He and Andrew shared an intense sexual experience, but nothing more. Lawrence finally saw how easily gay men can be tempted—and frustrated—by sexual play once they are given the chance (in this case, when he accepted Andrew's invitation to come up to his apartment). Sex is a wonderful thing, but a must for the conscious dater is to get to know a man before having sex.

As time went on, Lawrence found himself able to date men with less drama, and actually to have a good time during the process. He was no longer consumed with finding a man, and his desperation and neediness receded. As a result, after he met Santiago at a Gay Men's Chorus event and they dated a couple of times, though the relationship did not work out romantically, Santiago and Lawrence became good friends.

WHAT YOU'LL FIND IN THIS BOOK

My life experiences include working as a teacher, counselor, school principal, community activist, and, for the last decade, a dating and relationship coach within the gay community. As a coach, I have met thousands of gay men at my workshops throughout the United States. I love my work as a dating coach. I see men longing, at the deepest level, for an intimate, sensual, emotionally satisfying relationship. Not all gay men are just looking for sex. Gay men are no different than any other members of our society. We, too, have a powerful urge to create lasting partnerships.

One man was so keen on finding a man, he posted "WANTED" flyers around the city describing his assets and what he was after. Another man taped an open letter on a telephone pole, headed "I'm Available But Hate Singles Scene," and listing his harrowing experiences as a single man as well as how to reach him. I wouldn't suggest going to such lengths to find a man, but I do suggest that gay men ask themselves fundamental questions: Why do you want to date? What do you want to get out of dating? Perhaps you want more out of life, or something intrinsic seems missing. Freud said that, fundamentally, people are looking for happiness in two parts of their lives: love and work. Many men who come to see me are doing well in their careers, but their romantic life is lacking. Perhaps, for you, dating is a way of coming out—to yourself, about what you truly need.

Is dating a vehicle for broadening your social life? Some men develop their best friendships through dating. It is not uncommon for men to remain friends even after their romantic relationship ends. And I believe some gay men need to form deep friendships before they can move on to a steady boyfriend. These men—often isolated in high school and college—never learned the give-and-take of friendship, which forms the building blocks of more intimate relationships. It's vital that men sustain friendships over a period of time before they look for a partner for life.

Are you interested in raising a family? Today, you're likely to see gay couples with their kids at McDonald's or going to the playground together. Do you want to adopt, or find a surrogate mother?

Do you want to settle down? Do you see life passing faster than you could have imagined? When you hear "Carpe diem," does it suddenly mean more than it used to? Are you tired of living as a gay man perpetually in the fast lane?

It's not uncommon for men to tell me that they hope to grow old with someone. One man told me he wanted to share the seasons of life with a longtime companion. Some men feel an awakening inside, telling them to take more risks, to break out of their safe cocoons, really to embrace change.

So who is this book for?

- men who have just come out, men brand-new to the dating scene, and shy guys—men who need thorough, basic training in the fundamentals of dating

- men who date sporadically, but are not clear on what they want and need in another guy, or what they themselves bring to the dating table
- men who date a lot, but who have a history of meeting emotionally unavailable men and need a compass that will direct them to the best places to find a romantic partner
- men who are in the beginning stages of a relationship and need training in how to get along with their partner without self-sabotage
- men looking to move their relationship beyond the "taking it for granted" stage to a new level of soulful intimacy, one that challenges them to reveal more of who they are and to trust each other in the process

As a dating and relationship coach, I have had an incredible opportunity to see firsthand what ails the present gay-dating scene: men looking for the perfect body; guys not returning phone calls and performing disappearing acts; singles with attitude problems; and guys not being able to see past their penises. In this book, I address why it is so difficult for gay men to connect, and what prevents even the best and brightest among us from seeing our own strengths. I discuss how internalized homophobia can sabotage the best of intentions and thwart our search for true love. And I challenge all daters to throw out habitual patterns of self-judgment and perfectionism, making the case that one does not have to have the perfect body, to jeopardize his value system, or to lose his soul in his search for a boyfriend.

Dating is not rocket science. It is a skill that can be taught. And *Boyfriend 101* is intended to be practical, result-oriented, and—most of all—fun. I will teach you the technology of dating: the hows and wheres of meeting a mate, and what to do once you find him.

Boyfriend 101 should be useful to men all along the dating spectrum, from those who have just come out to those who are reentering the dating scene after a period away. As your coach, I'll be there for as you make your way through the dating world. Whatever your background and experience, I'll be in your corner, rooting for you.

For men with dating experience, I ask for a quick review of your personal history. Is your dating erratic and unfocused, as you wait for the right man to magically appear? Do you date on a regular basis, but meet only emotionally unavailable people? Take a look at the places you go to meet other singles and ask yourself if they really work for you. Perhaps you have the impulse to have sex too soon after you meet a guy, or you meet people online with no intention of taking the next step, of progressing from a virtual to an actual date.

What about your relationship history? Ask yourself, honestly, whether you find it difficult to maintain relationships beyond a few weeks or months. Facing tough situations—not always looking to bolt—is a sign of a mature dater. Let me show you the communications skills essential to any long-lasting, healthy relationship.

For those of you who have limited experience with dating, I ask that you consider the following questions:

- *Do you procrastinate about going out on dates?*
  "I have nothing to wear" . . . "I'll start dating next month" . . . "I've got to lose a few pounds first" . . .

- *Do you confuse getting laid and dating?*

  You have only one thing on your mind: s-e-x. "When and where can I get him into bed?"

- *Do you spend more time at the gym, Banana Republic, and Pottery Barn than you do with available singles?*

  You've become a slave to the gym and shopping. Dating is way down on your list of priorities.

- *Do you obsess about getting older and not finding a mate?*

  You live with the fear that there's not enough time and that the pool of available single men is dwindling.

- *Do you indulge in "rescue fantasy"—imagining "somebody will take care of me"?*

  For you, finding a man is like finding the magic bullet.

- *Are you obsessed with your body image?*

  You think your body is not perfect, that there's always something that needs to be improved.

- *Do you fear weekends, particularly Saturday nights?*

  Panic sets in and you'll do anything to avoid the pain of being home alone.

- *Do you like to talk about relationships as opposed to being in one?*

  You may indulge in relationship theory, but don't have a clue as to how to meet other guys.

- *Are you drinking too much and/or abusing drugs?*

  You find emotional comfort in the bottle, or that happiness depends on getting high.

- *Are you attracted to totally unavailable men?*

  This is certainly a way of not getting what you want and need, of forestalling happiness in your life.

• *Do you feel like an outsider in the gay community? Do you feel yourself inferior to other gay men?*

You may feel rebellious and angry toward the gay community, as well as abandoned.

If you answered yes to any of these questions, *Boyfriend 101* will help you take the right course of action. You may take baby or giant steps, but you'll take the steps no matter what, because your goal is very clear: to meet a man for a long-term relationship.

Dating, for most men, requires using a whole new set of muscles. As you work these muscles, you may hear moans and groans—your own. That's the sound of your dating life being born.

As you move through this book, you will develop many new skills that will provide a strong foundation for your dating life. You'll customize your own dating tool kit, filled with conversation builders, flirting techniques, and action plans—and then you can carry the tool kit anywhere, anytime, whether you're in a bar, a movie line, at a singles event, or vacationing in Provincetown.

You'll learn how to capitalize on strengths you didn't even know you possessed. You'll discover icebreakers that will enable you to start a conversation with ease. I will teach you how to find men who meet your needs, and how to gain or regain your confidence with other singles by knowing what to say and do on the first date. You'll learn how to negotiate safer sex. I'll discuss "types"—and offer practical tips for adding diversity to your dating experience by dating outside your type. You'll find the top 100 places to meet adorable men.

Boyfriend 101 may be challenging. That's my intention: to move you out of your comfort zone, so that you can see yourself and others from a new perspective.

Many of my client stories are based on composites, and—to respect confidentiality and maintain complete anonymity—all names have been changed. But you'll hear the real voices of real men, speaking the truth—from the gut—about themselves and the gay dating scene.

I am a prisoner of hope. I don't give up. I hope you won't, either. This book will provide a "dating map," to guide you on your journey: the adventure of your life! Stay the course.

My fondest wish is that you learn to be an inspiration to yourself, and become the ideal boyfriend.

BOYFRIEND 101

CHAPTER 1

GETTING STARTED

From the early days of Gay Liberation until the early 1980s, the primary place for meeting gay singles was bars. The bar scene was the hub of gay life. In bars, men dished, met new friends, fell in love, and broke up. Every gay traveler carried the *Damron Address Book,* the bible of gay travel. With the onset of AIDS in the early eighties, the golden age of bars ended. Suddenly, there were vastly more important things to do—ministering to others; taking care of one's own health—than hanging out in bars. With the decreasing importance of bars in the culture, new ways of relating emerged, as gay men sought alternatives to bars as places to socialize and to shelter themselves from the storm outside.

By the early 1990s, dating patterns for gay men had undergone a profound change. Previously, men met and either fell in love at first sight and became lovers fairly quickly, or had sex and, if it didn't work out, moved on. One rarely heard—let alone used—the "D" word. It sounded too straight. It took too much time. The expectation of immediately having sex with a man was so ingrained in gay culture that the idea of postponing what was only "natural" seemed old-fashioned and sex-phobic. To be gay was to have sex. Now.

The ritual of dating became a new phenomenon. New organizations sprang up across the United States, and gay community centers became an alternative hub of gay life, where one could meet other gay singles in a non-bar environment. Many men rubbed elbows with lesbians for the first time at gay centers, and experienced firsthand another model of same-sex coupling. Few lesbians were looking for the absolutely "perfect" body as much as gay men—or for immediate gratification.

Some men recoiled at the concept of dating, because they were afraid of intimacy—and still held on to the myth that the pre-AIDS period of sexual experimentation constituted the glory years. But those days are gone forever. The paradigm shift from bars, cruising, and immediate sex to dating, courtship, and long-term relationships defines today's gay landscape.

WHAT IS A DATE?

You're having a date when you meet a guy at a specified place and time in pursuit of the possibility of future romantic involvement. The operative words are *possibility* and *future;* throw the notion of immediate gratification out the window, because delayed gratification is part of the new paradigm.

Gay "dating" in the past was about immediacy, quickness, get-in-and-get-out, secrecy, fuck buddies, no commitments—there was always an exit. In no way do I condemn these patterns. Many gay men seized these opportunities as a means to explore their sexuality and to resist the heterosexist norms that had repressed them. No gay men wanted to be told what to do in bed or out of it.

The paradigm shift brought to gay singles the challenge of a new approach to intimacy. Learning how to date men, rather than just have sex with them, includes acknowledging and accessing what I call our "inner teenager." The inner teenager is the playful, shy, sexy, seductive, self-conscious, scared, and romantic part of us that wants to go out on dates, but may not possess the social and emotional skills to do it. There's a negative side to the inner teenager as well—the inner voices of temper tantrums. The adult part of us—the grown-up who can operate quite efficiently in the world—needs to take care of his inner teenager, or the inner teenager will rebel and make his life miserable.

Our inner teenager can make our career and work life seem like a death sentence if his needs don't get met. The inner teenager wants to come out and play, and requires the adult part of us to mentor him through the process. The inner teenager has a "dark" side that can tyrannize us and prompt us to act out on impulse.

Below are the voices of the inner teenager and—with mature responses—his adult:

TEENAGER: I'm afraid of asking him out.
ADULT: I'm going to call him this evening after work.

The inner teenager may appear cocky on the outside, but deep down inside he may lack the confidence and the social skills to ask a man out on a date. The inner teenager mumbles, fumbles, and makes everything a big deal. Being turned down becomes catastrophic.

Teenagers live with a heightened sense of reality; for them, everything is either "totally cool" or "totally bad." Adults need to provide balance, security, and perspective, and to de-escalate from all-or-nothing thinking. While the inner teenager is scared, the adult will show him that actions can be taken in spite of fear.

As an adult, you should find a comfortable place to make the call for a date: take a deep breath, dial the phone, and ask your guy out. Your inner teenager will be enormously appreciative!

TEENAGER: I want to get into shape.

ADULT: I'm going to watch my diet. I'm going to start working out, at least three times a week.

Teenagers can be undisciplined, so they need a lot of structure. A teenager may have a desire to get into shape, but McDonald's and Taco Bell may get in the way. Though the teenager may want to be king of the world, he is also very self-conscious about his body. The mature adult puts together a plan to get into shape, and sticks to it. The goal is to look great, on your own terms, so that your inner teenager can show off his body with confidence and pride.

TEENAGER: I'm scared he won't like me.

ADULT: I have a lot to offer him. I'm bringing a lot to the dating table.

The inner teenager is afraid of rejection. He wants to feel included and to have a sense of belonging. He feels all eyes are on him and doesn't want to "mess up." The adult in each single man must appreciate and acknowledge his assets and, like a peacock, strut his stuff to the world. The adult feels secure enough in himself not to take each rejection as a referendum on his value as a person.

TEENAGER: I want my dick sucked!
ADULT: When I do have sex, I make sure it's safe.

A teenager's raging hormones produce an enormous sexual appetite that insists on being satisfied. Some teenagers will have sex anytime, with anyone, throwing caution to the wind. They don't think about safe—or safer—sex. The adult must take care of his inner teenager by promising safe sex—and by proving that safer sex can make him happy.

TEENAGER: I want what I want, and I want it now!
ADULT: I need to understand that dating takes time. I'm not going to rush things.

Some teenagers have poor impulse control and find it quite difficult to delay gratification. Putting off short-term pleasure for a long-term goal is anathema to many young people. They want to see results yesterday. The grown-up gay man must temper his inner teenager's desire for immediate pleasure by setting realistic dating goals—for instance, going on as few as three dates per month. The grown-up can promise his inner teenager that he will meet some wonderful men, but must explain that it will likely take time, patience, and persistence.

Embrace the inner teenager—both his positive and negative sides. He needs to be told what to do in a sensitive way—gently, but sometimes firmly.

Remember that the adult is in charge—that if the inner teenager takes charge, he arrests your development. But if the inner teenager is totally denied, you may become a repressed and isolated man, losing the will to risk and live. The adult who encourages the positive in the inner teenager will celebrate and love the inner child who wants to come out and play.

A GAY RITE OF PASSAGE

There is a unique queer-developmental stage that most gay men must go through before accessing their inner teenager—colloquially, the slut stage; or, more demurely, the gay rite of passage. Gay men cannot discover their inner teenager and integrate him into their life until they pass through this gay rite of passage. Many straight boys can "sow their wild oats" without being judged; often, they are looked upon as exhibiting normal, healthy development. Many gay adolescents, though, have had to stifle their sexuality totally or to be secretive about what they have done and with whom, in order to avoid societal stigma or censure—sometimes even violence.

The gay rite of passage is a natural part of growing up gay and coming out completely as a gay man. This passage can take place during the early or late twenties, the thirties, the forties, or even later. Some men don't even realize they've gone through their gay rite of passage until years later.

Keith, thirty-six, spent fifteen years in an ashram as a celibate, and then arrived in San Francisco with barely a thousand dollars to his name. He shared an apartment with two other men, got a job at a local bookstore, and started to visit the Castro, meet guys, and have sex. He was never into public sex (backrooms, tearooms), preferring a warm bed instead. His sexual appetite astounded him: he never seemed to get enough. Keith enjoyed every moment of his gay rite of passage. He was slowly shedding his ethereal, sweet, "yoga boy" image, and was delighting in his newfound sexual freedom. But after about a year of his sexual dalliances, Keith was totally exhausted, and he announced to his friends that his period of sexual experimentation was coming to an end. He met Anthony, a massage therapist, at a yoga conference. They immediately hit it off, and began dating steadily.

It's important that gay men not feel guilty about such a rite of passage, and that they enjoy it while it lasts. Sex is as natural as eating—if we didn't eat, we'd starve, and sex-deprivation can starve us emotionally. (If you're from a religious tradition that is homophobic and sex-negative, I suggest you find a spiritual path that affirms your gay sexuality. Your other option is to stay within your religious group and fight for change, but this can be very problematic if you're dealing with entrenched, dogmatic beliefs.)

From my observation, the gay rite of passage lasts from six months to two years for most gay men. At some point, gay men intuitively know that it's over: "Been there—done that—now I need to move on to find a *man*." Remember, it's a developmental stage. Moving beyond the rite of passage is part of growing up. (The rite is not a way of life. You're not looking for tenure.) The gay rite of passage has ended when a man has integrated his sexuality into his dating and love life, and embraced his inner teenager.

Men stuck in the slut stage may have intimacy issues, or may be sexually compulsive, or may be terrified by the thought of dating. Intimacy issues can be dealt with in one-on-one or group therapy sessions. Sexually addicted men may choose to do sexual recovery through SCA—Sexual Compulsives Anonymous—in order to stop "acting out" and to develop a customized plan of healthier sexuality. As for men who are terrified of dating: I suggest they read this book from cover to cover!

TEN MYTHS OF DATING

Gay culture is rife with myths about gay dating patterns that just aren't true. Myths can take on a life of their own. One gay man says, "All men with blond hair are bottoms," and Joe in Chicago repeats it to his friend Rob in Boston. Thus, a myth is born. Soon, gay men everywhere begin to believe that all men with blond hair are bottoms, without any real evidence to back it up.

"Myth" is a nice word for misinformation. If not addressed, dating myths, at best, confuse the average dater, and, at worst, distort reality.

Myth #1: All the Good Guys Are Taken

Peter came to my Christmas workshop, "I Saw Michael Kissing Santa Claus." He's a six-foot-tall yoga teacher who is studying to be an interfaith minister. A pleasant man with beautiful blue eyes, Peter is friendly, but a bit shy. Still, I think he's a good catch. When I asked the guys to break up into groups of four to discuss desirable internal and external qualities, I noticed Peter looked a little lost, unable to find a group to hook up with. He said he was feeling really nervous. I told him to, at least, introduce himself to the men in the group.

I met Peter a month after the workshop, and he was dating Bill—a man from that group. He loved what Bill had said that night, and it had given him the confidence to share his thoughts and feelings. The two exchanged numbers and, shortly, started dating. Two beautiful souls—Peter and Bill—unexpectedly hooked up. These guys were not taken, and they were available for love!

When a gay man says all the good guys are taken, he's giving his power away. Men who don't want to take responsibility for their own dating life, preferring to live as the eternal, whiny victim—or, shall we say, the tragic queen—will never find happiness.

And what does it say about a gay man's self-esteem when he knows he's available but still believes this myth? Does he think he's not a "good guy"? Why would a gay single devalue himself so much? I believe it's because many gay men don't acknowledge or appreciate their own qualities. They think *everyone* out there is better than they are, and that's not true, either.

Myth #2: Dating Is Easy

Donald, a thirty-three-year-old computer programmer, works long hours at his job, sometimes sixty-hour weeks. He entered the dating scene hoping it would be easy, and it wasn't. We set up a dating schedule for him, blocking out time each week for "dating and fun."

The myth that dating is easy supports the assumption that "I don't have to take any action; I can sit in my rocking chair on the front porch and wait for someone to come to me." I know men who love their jobs/careers and men who hate their jobs/careers. You don't have to love dating to succeed, but you must be open to it, and you have to recognize that there is work involved.

I believe the work of dating is more about emotional than hands-on stuff. That's why there must be some payoff to dating—

and I don't mean sexual. With work, you get a check—a nice one, one hopes. With dating, is the payoff the fun of meeting new guys over a drink at the local bar? Is it going to a club for dancing? Is it the pleasure of joining a gay sports team?

Carl Jung said that when we take an action, there must be some positive payoff down the line or the subconscious will sabotage future action. I know guys who go on lots of dates, but they never seem to have any fun. Each date seems like a job interview, and is about as pleasurable as a root canal. Remember, dating might not be easy, but it ought to be fun!

Myth #3: Men Will Flock to Me for Dates

Dennis broke up with a lover of nine years, amicably. Dennis had never dated. He had met Christopher at a fund-raiser when he was twenty-seven, and they had immediately become a couple. So Dennis was angry when he found himself having to join the hunt for a boyfriend. He thought men would come to him without his doing anything.

If you're waiting for your prince to come, the length of the wait may surprise you. Ninety percent of men are not going to approach you—you're going to have to approach them. Even gorgeous guys need to make the first move.

I know it's humbling. But dating is not for divas.

Myth #4: Everyone in a Relationship Is Happy

A man sits in a café in West Hollywood, watching the happy couples walking by—hand in hand, smiling, not a care in the world—and he says to himself, "Why not me? Why can't I have that?"

Take it easy. There's a good chance you will meet some-one; but, in the interim, don't assume everyone in a relationship is happy. I can assure you there are some unhappy couples—straight and gay—whose members would prefer to be single. So enjoy your singlehood while it lasts.

We have such a single-phobic society that sometimes it seems that to be single is a fate worse than death. This puts pressure on singles to get into a relationship—any kind, as long as they're paired off. Better to wait for something right.

Myth #5: You Have to Look Like Tom Cruise to Get a Date

Chad, a twenty-seven-year-old editor, looks like Tom Cruise and doesn't even know it. He has a very high ideal—like so many gay men—of what beauty is in another man. Chad tells me that there are other men out there who are much better-looking than he. I tell him that there will always be men he will consider better-looking than himself. The trick—for Chad or anyone—is having enough confidence in your own appearance that you don't obsess over the appearance of others.

Ultimately, though, beauty is in the eye of the beholder, and I confess that, just like you, I've seen couples and wondered, "What does he see in *him*?" Advertising has done a number on all of us by presenting perfect Adonis images as the norm in gay life. That is not the norm. Stop seeing yourself as falling short of an unattainable ideal. It only keeps you from meeting some terrific men who don't fit the beauty myth.

And don't use "I'm not beautiful enough" as a defense against achieving real intimacy in your life. If you need to get into better shape, do so, but don't let the rigidity of the beauty myth keep you stuck with low self-esteem and isolation. Allow yourself to *discover* men instead of limiting yourself to preconceived notions of your type.

If you see a man who is impeccably dressed, you may say,

"He's out of my league." What league does he belong to? Go up and introduce yourself! You may discover he is more than his externals. And if you see a man who's in pretty good shape, except that he has a small paunch, allow yourself the possibility of seeing beyond the abdomen. He may have some other incredible attributes. Discover them. Discover *him*.

Myth #6: Older/Younger Relationships Don't Work

Kerry is a fifty-five-year-old professor who met his partner, Sean—who is twenty years younger—while searching the personal profiles on AOL. Kerry likes younger men for their energy, and Sean loves the stability of older men. They communicated through e-mail for about a month, and found they had much in common: both loved classical literature and music, the opera, and cooking; and both were more homebodies than travelers. Once they met, Kerry and Sean became inseparable.

Kerry is financially secure, and Sean—a music teacher at a private school, who gives piano lessons after school—makes only an average salary. One thing that concerned Kerry initially was whether Sean would be there for him as he got older. They both promised in their commitment ceremony (which was held two years after they met) to stay together "till death do us part." Sean's youth gave Kerry a life force which made him feel like a teenager. Kerry gave Sean the security he had craved since growing up in a working-class family preoccupied with money worries.

Kerry and Sean are an example of a successful cross-generational relationship. Each knew what he needed in another man and went after it. Now, if you're not into older or younger men, that is perfectly okay; but I ask all men not to set up any unnecessary barriers to meeting guys—maintain an open attitude. Some men adore the life experiences, loyalty, gentleness, and physical beauty of older men. Some older men love the energy, good looks, and spontaneity of younger guys.

Two stereotypes about cross-generational dating are worth considering—namely, the "trophy boyfriend" and the "sugar daddy." These are both fantasies, and fantasies don't hold a *healthy* relationship together. The trophy boyfriend, for someone with poor values, becomes nothing more than a commodity—like owning a Lexus, a *thing* to be consumed. And the sugar daddy becomes merely a means to an end. Eventually, there's a price to be paid for living out such fantasies.

However: if an affluent man has the desire to protect, take care of, and share his wealth with another man, and, on top of that, brings *other* attributes to the relationship besides his money, this, indeed, can form the basis for a healthy relationship. And if a man brings—*besides* his beauty—other qualities he can share with an older mate, that, certainly, is okay, too. As long as both are honest—with themselves and with each other—about what they're doing.

Myth #7: I Can't Deal with Rejection

Diego attended my workshop "Shy Guys Are Tops!" and asked me a question in front of the group: "How do you deal with rejection? I can deal with just about anything in life but getting turned down." The whole room went dead quiet. I, too, heard such sadness in his voice, I felt an impulse to respect it with silence. But I knew I could not do that. I have to be honest with my clients, and tell them that rejection goes with the territory. You'll drive yourself up the wall if you let rejection possess you, and clutter up your mind with "I'm not worthy" chatter.

Rejection has more sting when we put all our eggs in one

basket—latching on to one guy instead of playing the field. Dating is an adventure on which you can meet many men.

Of course, rejection takes on added weight when we've been intimate—have shared a deep part of ourselves—and then get that awful call: "I like you but I don't think there's a match." This can cause anyone to go temporarily insane. So be conscious and careful of whom you have sex with, and of the emotional consequences.

Ultimately, though, the best answer to rejection is a four-letter word: "Next!"

Myth #8: Internet Matchmaking Services Don't Work

A client I saw on a regular basis was working on his dating action plan and came upon a matchmaking service that gave subscribers three categories from which they could meet men: for friendship, for romance, or for sex. The client chose romance and friendship, since he didn't want to get distracted by one-night stands. Over the course of three months, he met ten men, and one of those men became his partner. I remember my client sheepishly revealing to me that he had met someone and that, therefore, he wouldn't need my services anymore. I was ecstatic, and told him that the purpose of our work was for him to meet a mate and move on!

Nothing is absolute in the dating game. Some things work. Some don't. Matchmaking services can provide an enormous service for men who need an extra push to get the ball rolling. There is a feast of men from all walks of life you can discover through these services.

Myth #9: Dating Is Not Fun

Though dating requires work, it has to be fun; otherwise, we'll never be motivated to take a risk.

Robert is a focused professional who takes work very seriously, so he wanted to meet a man quickly, with little trouble. Throughout his sessions with me, he performed all the tasks in his dating action plan religiously, and usually asked what else he could do to achieve his goal of finding a man. He would take copious notes during each session, as if he were sitting through a lecture. During our fifth session together, I told him he needed to relax a bit.

So we made a list of places where he could be silly, have fun, and possibly find a man to date. He started going to a cabaret bar each Thursday, and he joined a salsa dance group. Once Robert began to sit back and enjoy the ride, he found himself opening up to more people, and he felt more confident about himself.

You can keep dating fun by not focusing on the outcome—"Will he or won't he be my future husband?"—and, instead, staying "in the moment" with your date. Suggest to your date fun places to go (an amusement park, a wrestling competition) and to do (drive to the ocean, go horseback riding). Stop seeing a date as a talkathon in which each man spills his guts for an hour or two! You can talk *and* have fun at the same time.

Some other fun and/or quirky things to do on a date:

- go bowling
- go surfing
- do yoga
- go to a drag show
- get spa treatments

Myth #10: Successful People Have an Easier Time Dating

I work with successful people, and they have the same struggles as common folk. Dating is a great equalizer.

Mitch is forty-two, works in real estate, and has incredible verbal dexterity. When he came to see me, I said to myself, "Why is he here? He's so outgoing!" Mitch told me that he had been in a fifteen-year relationship, which had broken up two years before, and that he didn't know where to meet guys. As he spoke, he seemed increasingly vulnerable, and I could see that he was still feeling significant sadness over his breakup. He was alone and wanted to share his life with someone special.

Mitch knew he had a lot to offer another man. His courage in seeking out coaching was a giant step toward admitting that, despite his success in life, he needed help just like other men.

THE DATING SPECTRUM

We don't want to be ruled by the tyranny of myths or tales from the dating world. They restrict us and keep us stuck in a negative belief system. They certainly don't get our energy going. Let's leave the myths behind us to take a look at the dating spectrum and where you, as a gay single, fit into it.

Part of a man's self-assessment is to know his place along the dating spectrum. The spectrum encompasses the full range of possibilities: from the beginner who's taking tentative steps out of the closet to the more experienced man, who may already have one or more long-term relationships under his belt.

The dating law of physics states: absolutely no one is in the same place at the same time in the dating scene—some men may know precisely where they're at; some may be in a fog, or in denial, or are ashamed to know their place. But knowing where you're at will help you determine the steps you need to take in order to achieve your goal of finding new love in your life.

In the Closet

Shelby, an African American from Baltimore, decided to come out at forty-two, a major step for a man from a very close-knit family whose belief system denied black men could be gay. Shelby couldn't take the closet any longer. Having sex with escorts and going home with strangers from bars at two in the morning no longer had any appeal. Attending a political symposium sponsored by gay activists at the local university, he was astounded by the caliber of men he found there and made a conscious decision to come out to his family and friends, even though it was going to be excruciatingly difficult. Shelby found a gay therapist and began the process.

Closeted men lead compartmentalized lives based on secrecy and shame, and it's challenging to be in a healthy, mature relationship with them. Most of us have been in the closet—some longer than others—and we know how stifling and claustrophobic a world it can be. In the closet, we are never at our best, and we're never really at ease. Formerly closeted men have told me how much they lied to family and friends about who they were seeing. ("We're really only good friends." "We're going off camping with some friends.") One man told me he couldn't spend Thanksgiving with his newfound boyfriend because it wouldn't look right.

If someone wants to remain in the closet, that's his business, but I have to be frank with the men I work with and tell them that men who choose to stay in the closet are not emotionally available. For older men who are in the closet and afraid to come out, I suggest reading *Golden Men: The Power of Gay Midlife,* by Harold Kooden and Charles Flowers. I also suggest contacting one of the local gay/lesbian centers listed in the back of this book, and asking agencies within the center for available support groups for men coming out late in life.

When a man lives in fear of being gay, the worst thing is to remain isolated. He needs to be around other men to talk about his fears of and concerns about coming out. A supportive community is crucial to a healthy coming out.

Out but Never Dates

Lorenzo is out but never dates. He's thirty-eight and hasn't had a date in five years—lots of casual sexual encounters, but never a date. He felt totally embarrassed about this, so I told him that there are other gay men who have never been on a date in their lives, but are too ashamed to admit it.

As a dater, come clean. Wherever you're at is totally cool.

Sexually Addicted

Men who are acting out sexually may be going through their "slut stage," or they may have an addiction to sex. The difference between fucking for fun and pleasure, and sex addiction, is that the addictive mind has no built-in controls to stop having sex.

Mike came out when he was twenty-five, after going to graduate school on the West Coast. He moved back to Chicago and started going to clubs, and would take guys home to have sex on an average of three times a week. Then he began going to cruising areas for sex as well, and watching gay porn. Mike could never get enough, any time of the day. He began arriving at work late and calling in sick more than was usual. His friends didn't know where he was most of the time—they'd call and leave messages, and he'd call back when he knew they wouldn't be in, telling them he was working on a special project. Sex for Mike was no different than alcohol was for the alcoholic. Dating for Mike was an abstraction. He couldn't conceive of meeting a good-looking guy and not having sex.

Don't expect to date a man who is sexually compulsive. Sex addicts need help; they are not emotionally ready to date. However, through gradual, painstaking sexual recovery, many gay men have blossomed into fully functioning, available singles.

Dates Infrequently

There's another group of singles who date very infrequently—perhaps five times a year. These men may go to a dating service or put an ad in the paper, even meet guys, but get easily discouraged when things don't work out. They may experience rejection and need a lot of time to recoup. This group of daters may also include men who are very committed to their work and career, and have therefore put dating on the back burner. Such men go in and out of dating and never fully commit to the process.

The in-and-out daters make up a fairly large group of gay singles. I have found dating action plans to be very successful for this group, because plans keep them on track and out of the "Am I dating or am I not?" Twilight Zone. (A dating action plan generates concrete and specific actions customized to the needs of each individual. For instance, one man's plan may include getting calling cards made up and a new photo for online dating services, while another man's plan may include introducing himself to three people in a bar setting over the course of a week, and joining one gay sports club.)

Dates but Meets the Wrong Guys

Are you one of the singles who date the *wrong* guys? Do you keep asking yourself, "Why do certain men seem to come to me, and why do I seem to be attracted to them for only the first two dates?"

I believe that there are men who have the ability to make a very good impression on a first date, and who may even exude sexual energy, but who—after the second date—seem to morph into a variation on the "date from hell." One totally exasperated man told me, "I've spent so many years in therapy, and I still meet guys from planet Mars."

The "wrong" guys are always going to be out there. As you become a more aware dater, you'll be able to spot them sooner than later. Ask yourself: Does he listen to you on a date, or is he too self-involved? Is there exchange in conversation, or only his rambling monologues? Do you feel something in your gut that makes you uneasy about the guy? Does he obsess about sex, or ask you so many questions you feel you're being cross-examined?

When Mr. Wrong is staring you in the face, you need to tell him gracefully that you don't feel any chemistry, and move on to meeting other guys. Don't start describing his character defects to him or, worse, play therapist. It's not your job to fix him.

In Transition—from a Breakup or the Death of a Partner

Men in this group have been in a long-term relationship, but— due to a breakup or the passing of a partner—find themselves looking for a new mate. When one is used to living with someone now gone, there is a natural impulse to immediately fill the void—to want solace, comfort, security, companionship, and someone to sleep with. The pain of being by oneself is too unbearable for some of these men.

For such men, I recommend waiting at least six months to a year before dating. There must be time to grieve the loss of a relationship, and to get one's bearings; otherwise, one never lets go of the old, formerly shared, emotional life. And no one wants to date the "ghost" of a former partner. This period of adjustment requires the support of family and friends, not support from people you're dating.

In my work, I meet many men in transition, some of whom bring a great deal of positive relationship experience to the dating scene. Some of them are in their late thirties, forties, and fifties. They possess knowledge of the world, a certain detachment from drama, and an ability to listen to other people. They can "show up" for people when most needed.

To come to the dating scene when you're more "mature" can be quite humbling. It's like starting over; but, as I tell all seasoned men, there's one quality they bring to the dating scene that they're totally unaware of: they know that the perfect man doesn't exit. They are much less prone to fantasy—a good start! Though they certainly like a nice-looking man, more easily than men less tested by time they can focus on the internal qualities and values that another man possesses. "Being" with someone, as opposed to "being seen" with someone, takes precedence.

Dating Troupers

The real troupers of the dating scene date a lot of terrific guys, but have not yet found a partner. Some of these men think they are "always a bridesmaid, never a bride," but I tell them that they are men who simply have not met the right guy, and are willing to hang in there for the long haul, until they do—"sometimes a bridesmaid, one day a bride."

DATING SELF-ASSESSMENT

> This above all: to thine own self be true,
> And it must follow, as the night the day,
> Thou canst not then be false to any man.
>
> —WILLIAM SHAKESPEARE, *HAMLET*

We bring ourselves into the dating world. Before you begin dating, it's important to take stock of your relationship history and your gay social life. Use this section on dating assessment as an opportunity for self-inquiry and reflection. Consider the following questions:

How many long-term relationships (lasting at least one year) or short-term relationships have you had, and why/how did they end?
Having been in a long-term relationship does not necessarily earn you a gold star. If it was a healthy and fulfilling union, though, you do bring a big plus to future relationships.

Did your relationship end because you simply outgrew each other and needed to move on? (Some men's exes become their friends for life.)

Did your relationship end due to a unilateral communications breakdown, or did both of you share the responsibility?

Was it a long-term relationship—say, of five years' duration— that needed to end after six months; but, because you feared being alone, you became roommates posing to yourselves as lovers? (Some men can't fathom not being in a relationship. They reason that a warm body is better than no body, and end up jumping from one partner to another with no real clarity or understanding of why their relationships are not working.)

Do they leave you, or do you initiate breakups?

Some men—knowingly or unknowingly—always dump lovers after a short period of time. They may gain a distorted sense of power by doing this, but deep down, they are terrified of intimacy or even of getting what they need from another person.

When men have told me stories about guys who disappear with nary a word, I feel for them deeply, and beg them not to beat themselves up about it. At the same time, I ask them to determine whether there's any pattern of behavior in *themselves* that attracts such thoughtless men. (Some men, abandoned emotionally as children by their parents, suffer repetition compulsion: they unconsciously seek out men they think will love them but who will ultimately abandon them, just as their parents did. In such cases, I encourage therapy for help in dealing with abandonment issues and the propensity for meeting emotionally unavailable men.)

Are you addicted to chaos, thriving only when there is major drama in a relationship?

There is *always* some drama in relationships; but, when it becomes *high drama,* we need to pull back and observe the part we're playing. The story of Sam and Roger is illustrative of two well-intentioned people coming together and, eventually, learning some of the hard lessons of being in a relationship.

Sam, now forty-four, is an investment consultant who grew

up in an upper-middle-class family outside Memphis. Roger, thirty-eight, is an aspiring screenwriter living off a trust fund. After six years, Sam ended their relationship. They loved—and continue to love—each other, but could no longer be partners.

Roger is an active alcoholic, in and out of rehab centers for most of their partnership. Sam and Roger were classic codependents. Sam needed to take care of Roger—it gave him a sense of control. "Poor Roger" became more his child than an equal. Sam would clean up after him whenever Roger went on a bender; and, of course, Roger willingly played the bad boy. Each played into the other's negative qualities.

They were living in codependent heaven, oblivious of the "elephant in the middle of the room," until Sam started going to Al-Anon meetings and began to get a whole new perspective on the dynamic between Roger and himself—that what he saw as helping Roger was no more than enabling. Sam could not let Roger live his own life, or make his own mistakes and hit bottom, if necessary, in order to face his demons. Roger, of course, played into Sam's caretaking instinct by crying a lot, and recounting his miserable childhood.

When Sam did his self-assessment with me—and confessed his attraction to alcoholics and alcoholic behavior—he was able to state, emphatically, that he did not want to go out anymore with any alcoholic *not* in recovery, or to play a codependent role. A year after his breakup with Roger, Sam met Bertrand at a Gay Expo, and can now report that he has never felt better.

"I had no idea of what it meant to be in a sane and nurturing relationship. The chaos is gone. I'm impressed by how organized Bertrand is, and how terribly disorganized Roger and I were. We didn't balance our checkbooks. We would lose things. We were late for events."

Roger and Sam continue to be in touch. Roger broke his leg while in France, and Sam went over to see him—but established clear boundaries. (He stayed three days and came home.) There is still a little part inside Sam that wants to take care of Roger, but he now knows Roger has to grow up and take care of himself.

It's called detaching, with love.

How would you describe your life?

The life that you're leading now is the life you're bringing to the dating table. Can it be improved? Expanded? What are your interests, hobbies? What are your friends like? Do you belong to any social organizations, religious groups? What do you do on weekday nights, on weekends? Do you spend a lot of time by yourself, and is that out of choice or because you don't know how to—or are afraid to—meet new people? Can you say, without hesitation, that you have a passion for life?

During a self-assessment session, I asked Joey what his interests were, and for a second he looked dumbfounded—as if I had thrown him a curveball.

"I can't think of any. Well, I visit my mother every week. I meditate twice a week at the Zen center, and once a month I attend their all-day meditation session. I see my therapist once a week."

I told Joey that visiting his mother, meditating, and seeing his therapist were not the interests I was talking about, even though they were integral to his life.

I spoke to Joey about fun, asking, "What would you like to do for fun? What would you like to do but, for some reason, aren't able to do? Have you read about anything in a magazine or newspaper, or heard about something at work or from a friend, that would interest you?"

He thought for a moment, took a deep breath, and said, "This may sound stupid, but there's a gay bingo night at the gay center which I'd like to attend. Also, my friend Milton goes two-stepping and I'd like to learn that. And I've always wanted to learn how to swim!"

Within a month, Joey had played gay bingo, joined the two-steppers, and put his name on a waiting list at the local Y for swimming lessons. I also told him about gay aquatics, in which he might like to participate someday.

Joey began to develop interests and to cultivate a queer social life. These are very important assets he can bring to the dating table. (Now when a date asks what his interests are, he doesn't have to say, "I visit my mother"!)

Do you take part in gay culture?

Is your social life broad-based (encompassing museums, base-ball, and jazz clubs) or is it more gay-centered (primarily visiting the gay center, if there is one in your town or city; going to gay vacation spots; joining gay organizations; joining gyms that are either gay or gay-friendly; etc.)?

Earl told me he has a lot of interests and does lots of socializing, but most of the time it's outside the gay community. He loves baseball and goes to Fenway Park as much as he can, with straight friends (who know he's gay). He belongs to a bowling club that grew out of the housing complex he lives in, and he's a member of the local Green Thumb organization, which spends Saturday mornings sprucing up community gardens.

I asked Earl if he would like to engage in some gay-related activities around Boston, and he said "Sure" but didn't know where to go. For starters, I told him about the Beantown Softball

League and the Chiltern Mountain Club, which has great out-door activities and sponsors weekends out of town. Earl heard that Chiltern was doing a weekend away in May, so he decided to take the plunge and enter the world of the gay outdoors.

Do you have financial limitations that make dating difficult?

Dating does require some money, but you don't have to be well-off to date. I recommend being up front about what your budget is when you meet and make a date with someone. You can always say, "Things are a little tight right now so I have to do cheap for a while." If a guy really likes you, and money is not one of his top priorities, he will understand.

Besides, there are lots of ways to have fun without spending a fortune. You can cook a nice meal at home cheaply. You can go to parks, or look for cultural events that are free or cost very little.

Is the fear of AIDS holding you back?

Are you fearful of contracting HIV, or are you concerned about passing the virus along to someone else? Talking about HIV issues with someone at your local AIDS organization is crucial to overcoming these fears. HIV will be with us for a very long time. Single gay men must become comfortable with discussing HIV, and not let it limit or take away the joy of life.

Do you think you're out of the dating loop because of your age?

Many gay men feel their chance of meeting someone diminishes after forty-five (if not sooner!), which can easily become a self-fulfilling prophecy. There is a Talmudic saying that covers this: "We do not see the world as it is but as we are." If a single man sees himself as too old to be in the dating loop, he may project his attitude that "there's no one out there for me" onto others, limiting his possibilities. But if an older guy sees himself as smart and good-looking, and he possesses other great qualities—including his belief in himself—his chances of meeting men increase.

WHAT I BRING TO THE DATING TABLE

The first part of your dating self-assessment involved taking a look at your relationship history and your gay social life. The next step in the self-assessment is to examine your internal and external qualities, so you know what you bring to the dating table.

External Qualities

In my experience with gay men in workshop settings and during one-on-one consultations, most gay men find it much easier to list their internal qualities (sensitivity, loyalty, etc.) than their external qualities (nice physique, beautiful eyes, and so forth). With all the perceived emphasis on the externals in gay culture, you would think it would be just the opposite. It isn't. Why?

Many gay men, on the surface, may seem as if they like their bodies; but, deep down, they see only a flawed human being needing vast improvement. They are quite skilled at *presenting* themselves to the world, but the search for validation seems never-ending, and the more they search for it the more self-conscious they become. Some men simply cannot say, "I have a warm smile" or "My pecs look great in a white T-shirt."

Gay men need to acknowledge their external qualities, not in an arrogant or in-your-face way (that's vanity), but with an easy-going self-confidence. Recognizing our external qualities is not about one-upmanship or making ourselves feel superior at the expense of others. Our beauty is a gift to be shared with other human beings.

External qualities also encompass skills (carpentry, cooking), achievements (outstanding figure skater), and talents (singing, playing an instrument). Think about the external qualities that you bring to the table. Don't worry if you're not sure if a particular attribute is an internal or an external quality. To help you get started, here is a list of external qualities you can choose from and/or add to. (Remember: be imaginative.)

great teeth	crossword puzzle fanatic
handsome face	nice nose
fantastic swimmer	cute butt
excellent gardener	great hiker
accomplished musician/artist	dedicated yachtsman
scholarly historian	own my own business
fine fiction writer	ran the marathon
appreciate antique furniture	great dancer
committed to working out	raised two children
do a lot of volunteer work	speak three languages
budding screenwriter	won two wrestling contests
sense of humor	S/M activist
dedicated teacher	great at magic tricks
soccer coach	

Internal Qualities

Naming internal qualities is a lot easier for gay men than naming external qualities, though certainly not for all of us. Internal qualities characterize the emotional life of the dating scene. They are qualities deep inside you—in your belly, in your heart. They are soulful and long-standing. Internal qualities survive time. They are the qualities you will need as you grow old with your partner.

Honesty

I asked Harry what internal qualities he can bring to another man. He thought for a moment and said, "I'm a good person. I don't cheat. I pay my taxes. I think I try to give people the benefit of the doubt." Smart, attractive, and ambitious, Harry brings the internal quality of honesty to the dating world.

Warmth

Avi possesses the internal quality of warmth. His smile lights up a room. People like being around him. He's a cranial-sacral massage therapist, and people flock to him for his service. One person observed about Avi, "After being in his presence you always feel a lot better about yourself."

Confidence

Whether hang-gliding, competing in bike marathons, or speaking in front of groups, Tim exudes a natural confidence that makes him a very appealing guy to other singles. He's self-assured and cocky, but not obnoxious and overbearing. People like Tim's energy. They don't resent him.

Stability

Josh, forty-four, a stock analyst, is a solid and steady individual whom people depend on when things get rough. "Josh, I have a real problem here. Do you have time for coffee?" Josh shows up for people. There's an inner strength that comes across, along with a keen sense of humor.

Nurturing

Roberto is a thirty-four-year-old small-business owner who has the capacity to nurture other people. Roberto's quality of taking care of someone (as long as the caretaking is mutual) is a real gift, and anyone who has this quality should not be taken for granted. As you get a little older and more wise, I promise you will value nurturing in a partner more than anything.

Positive outlook

Martin, thirty-four, has been working as an interfaith minister for three years. His spirituality is based on affirming and believing the positive in life without denying the negative. As with Avi, people like being around Martin. His positive outlook on life is contagious.

Intuitive

The derivation of the word *intuition* is "to look at or contemplate." Kirk, twenty-nine, an avid soccer player, is by nature very intuitive. He has a highly prized gift of "reading" people and sensing what they're about without being arrogant or invasive. In the dating world, Kirk's intuition is very practical, since he can "sense" things about a man and make some fairly quick evaluations based on his intuition.

Now, just as you did with external qualities, I want you to think about all the internal qualities you can offer another man. Feel free to expand upon this list:

innerly peaceful	childlike
balanced	thoughtful
self-reliant	sincere
resilient	inner-directed
committed	determined
persevering	creative
joyful	spiritual
serious-minded	

Remember: don't be stingy with yourself, or afraid to tell others what you have to offer. I know many, many men who have enormous gifts, but are too reticent about showing them to the world. As you grow more confident in acknowledging your pluses, you'll see other gay men from a fresh perspective. You'll want to *share* your qualities and gifts with another man.

Why hold on to them? Life is too short. Love is waiting for you around the corner. Use your inventory of internal and external qualities as a springboard toward finding the love you want.

WANTS VS. NEEDS

For the first time in my life I was really aware of another person's body, of another person's smell. We had our arms around each other. It was like holding in my hand some rare, exhausted, nearly doomed bird which I had miraculously happened to find.

—JAMES BALDWIN, *GIOVANNI'S ROOM*

Knowing what we want in a relationship and which of our needs must be met by it is an important development for any dating man. Without this knowledge, we are doomed to date men who will only cause us pain and grief.

In his first coaching session, Larry—a twenty-nine-year-old small-business owner—was practically screaming, "These guys don't know what they want!" He was totally irritated by the men he encountered in the dating world. "I met this guy George, and we went out on five dates. We got along fine. We drank, danced, talked for hours, and discovered a lot we had in common—both native Californians who grew up in middle-class families, got involved in politics, and loved New York City. We had fantastic sex on the fourth date and went out for dinner on the fifth date. I called George a couple of times after that, and he didn't respond. I got worried, thinking something might have happened to him. I waited another day, and then e-mailed him that I was trying to reach him and wanted to know if he was okay. I got an e-mail back which I read in total disbelief: in a nutshell, he told me he was confused about our relationship, and wasn't sure whether I was the right person for him. He really liked me, and felt very close during sex, but he wasn't sure what he wanted in a man. And then he wrote, 'Talk to you soon.' "

I told Larry he had every right to scream. It can be pretty frustrating for a man with the best of intentions to comprehend why other singles can't get their act together. Larry had worked hard to get where he was. Like so many other gay singles, he wonders whether he will ever meet a man with drive, focus, and ambition like his.

How many men say they only want to date men who are *serious* about relationships, but have little gravitas themselves? How many men have been seduced by the hope that the perfect single man will just suddenly appear in their lives, even when they haven't considered what "perfection" for them might be? Why does it seem so many gay singles have no idea what they're looking for, as they bounce from one fantasy of a lover to another?

I meet all sorts of men who—whether twenty-six, thirty-four, or forty-five—simply *don't know what they really want* in a guy. They've been conditioned by a slick, youth-obsessed media and limit their wants to an airbrushed man who exists only in digitized form. Some straight men I have spoken to will see an image of an impossibly beautiful woman and then make love to their girlfriends with the memory of that beauty in mind. Far too many gay men see a fantastic body and imagine that's what they must have in a partner.

A *want* is a strong desire; a *need* is a physiological or psychological requirement for our well-being. My thesis is that if you give gay men an opportunity to explore all of their wants, they can then winnow them down to basic needs or "requirements." I conduct "wants vs. needs" exercises in my private consultations and at my public seminars. These exercises have proven to be very effective in helping men explore and focus on their wants and needs. The purpose of such an exercise is to tap into the deepest part of a man's emotional life, which may have remained dormant for many years. The man then has a chance to discover what he has repressed or denied, or what the wants and needs are that he dare not admit to himself.

I suggest that you make a list of what you want in a mate, organized into categories: intellectual, emotional, social, financial, physical, spiritual, value-based, sexual/sensual, cultural, and specifics that are particularly important to you. Some of these considerations may be more important to you than others; for instance, your emotional wants may far exceed your cultural wants. Each reader's list will be as different as their fingerprints. There are no "right" answers, only truthful responses.

Intellectual

An intellectual value is one that appeals to our mind. Are we stimulated by this man in conversation? Are we challenged by his ideas? Is finding a man with a similar educational background to yours important or not? Do you value an inquiring mind? Is it important to you that your man think things through before taking an action? Do you enjoy a good debate? Do you like voracious readers, guys who speak many languages, men who approach the *Times* crossword with devotional fervor and complete it in ink?

Consider two men who have totally different views on getting, intellectually, what they want in a man. Neither is better than the other. They are just different.

Gordon is a psychotherapist and fiction writer who enjoys nothing more than gabbing about books (fiction and nonfiction) and characters (real or imaginary). For Gordon, intellectual wants are a top priority in a date and potential mate. This does not mean that Gordon believes he is superior or even highbrow, only that he knows what he wants and is honest enough to admit it.

Carl went to the Wharton School of business and, unsurprisingly, has a keen business sense. He met Brendan, a bartender, and—attracted to Brendan's cockiness and lust for life—didn't feel it important to be stimulated intellectually by him. Going to a baseball game, visiting Brendan's family, renovating their country house, and watching TV are the things Carl treasures in this relationship. Carl is not "settling." Connecting with Brendan has helped him get a new perspective on life. He can be intellectual at work, but when it comes to his love life, Carl likes a man who is down-to-earth.

Emotional

Emotional wants are key to any healthy relationship. Is it important for you to have a man "show up" for you when things get rough? Is his capacity to nurture important? What about being able to provide sound advice, or listen to you, or share a safe space of emotional intimacy? Is it important that you bring out the best in each other, value each other, feel safe and protected together? Is moving in with someone a high priority for you, or do you prefer your own space?

Important as emotional wants are to all relationships, they may be more so for men who gravitate to the role of caretaker or those for whom a relationship is a source of stability. For Matthew—a thirty-three-year-old who never knew his dad, and whose mother died when he was nineteen—feeling safe and protected in a relationship ranked high on the list of emotional wants. Matthew—always attracted to men ten or more years his senior—met Hugh, a forty-six-year-old psychologist, at a Gay Men's Chorus fund-raiser. Hugh is very nurturing and protective of Matthew without being overbearing. For example, when Matthew was going through a job change and needed to revise his résumé, Hugh offered a Sunday afternoon to help, and even to go over some possible interview questions. Matthew always finds Hugh's advice and counsel indispensable; in turn, Matthew provides Hugh with welcome care, including back massages and home-cooked dinners. He also loves to hear Hugh play the piano, and accompanies him to his monthly piano recitals at the local Episcopalian church.

Consider what you want in a man emotionally. Is trusting your partner to be committed to a monogamous relationship important to you? Is getting good advice and counsel? Is it important that you're able to fight fair and openly disagree, without feeling that the roof is going to cave in at any moment? Do you like it when a man compliments you, reassures you, and has the capacity to hold your hand through the darker moments of life? Does a man meet your emotional wants when he is playful, when he surprises you with special gifts, when he smiles on seeing you, when he tells you directly that you mean a lot to him?

Social

What do you want in a man socially? Is it important that he like to go dancing and take tango lessons at the Y? Go to basketball games? Play poker with friends? Enjoy large dinner parties? Visit his family or yours? Go double-dating?

Bradley, thirty-five, owns a florist shop and loves to throw big, lavish dinner parties. He wanted a man who enjoyed his Auntie Mame spirit, but his former boyfriend didn't appreciate these parties and thought them a waste of time and money, so they fought a lot. Bradley didn't share with his ex, in the beginning of their relationship, what these social home gatherings mean to him. Lesson learned: be honest with your man-to-be about what you want, from the start.

Financial

Financial wants bring up big issues for gay men. Most men find it easier to talk about dick size than finances. So ask yourself: Am I wrong for wanting a man who is rich? Am I still a liberal Democrat if I want a man who earns more than $75,000 a year? Is it important that my man not be in debt? What about the size of his portfolio? Can I be attracted to a man who lives a simple life, who earns and spends little money but seems to be content? Do I want a man who can perform the simple task of balancing his checkbook? A man who isn't secretive about money?

Nathaniel, fifty-five, is a wealthy businessman who doesn't care how much a man makes as long as he has a job and goes to work every day. Nathaniel could be a good provider, but he doesn't want to earn the sobriquet "sugar daddy." He wants a man who will ask him, when he comes through the door, "How was your day?" Someone who can talk about his business for twenty minutes or so over a martini, someone who really listens to him. It is imperative to Nathaniel that the man he meets not feel financially beholden to him.

If Nathaniel does find a man who earns far less than he does, his good intentions may work well for the first few months of the relationship, when everything seems like heaven, but as people really get to know each other, intentions and motivations become a lot clearer. When there is disparity in income, both parties must talk about this issue sooner rather than later, and the basic ground rule for this discussion is that both men come to the table as equals, regardless of their financial standing. Once they've reached a clear understanding, Nathaniel may give his future partner a trip to Key West as a Christmas gift, and his partner may plan an overnight camping trip to the state park, "all expenses paid," without misunderstanding on either side. As long as both men proceed openly, honestly, and from the heart, the disparity of income will not be problematic. If this healthy attitude is not present, resentment, suspicion, and even paranoia might well destroy the relationship, despite the best of intentions.

Harvey—a social worker with a job at a high school and a part-time therapy practice—had spent five years in a Zen monastery. Money was not a big priority for Harvey. His tastes were simple, and he wanted to meet an "ordinary guy." Recently, he had a commitment ceremony with Jeff, who works for the U.S. Postal Service. They are doing extremely well as a couple.

Harvey and Jeff seem to share similar values regarding money, and I believe this will help their relationship. They have joint checking and credit-card accounts for day-to-day household expenses, which Harvey enters weekly into the computer, listing shared expenses very clearly (food, telephone, electricity, cable), as distinct from personal expenses, for which each partner has his own checking account and credit card (cell phone, theater, dining out alone, etc.). They have an excellent accountant to help them with the everyday financial issues, as well as manage their investments.

Dean, thirty-three, is an investment banker. When I asked him what he wanted in a man, financially, he didn't hesitate: "a man who makes, at least, a hundred thousand a year." It was clear that, for Dean, there must be some equality in earning. Of course, Dean is limiting his pool of men with his hundred-thousand minimum. I never try to persuade a client to change their wants, but I did say to Dean, "Many good men don't make a hundred thousand dollars." He said, "I must have a guy who's an equal, or who makes more money than I do. That's the way I think."

Physical

In the past, some gay men focused entirely on the physical when they evaluated a man. Though the physical still has enormous weight in the gay community, it's getting some competition these days from other attributes.

Still, you need to know: What do you want in a man, physically? Do you want a man who is muscular? Slender? Washboard stomached? Big-bellied? Dark featured? Stocky? Tall? With a bubble butt? Broad shoulders? Great teeth? A nice smile?

You may get a bit self-conscious when asked to verbalize what you want physically in a man. But don't edit anything out. Feel free to express your wants without shame or embarrassment. Have fun with the physical! Let's enjoy the human body with all its shapes and contours, perfections and imperfections.

Spiritual

Over the years, spirituality has become a much higher priority for gay men than previously. Spirituality does not necessarily mean adherence to a particular religion. Many gay men have been tortured psychologically by organized religions with homophobic messages.

During the late eighties and nineties, an incredible number of gay spiritual groups were created in an attempt to satisfy the deep spiritual thirst that many gay people have. My friend Tom met his partner at a gathering of the Radical Faeries, a pagan-influenced spiritual group. Tom, a retired Catholic, was searching for a spiritual connection and liked the free spirit and community of the Faeries.

Esteban, a twenty-six-year-old personal trainer who isn't Jewish, started going to classes about the kabbalah (part of the Judaic mystical tradition), and met some great guys who were committed to a spiritual path. He started dating a Jewish guy, Brian, and the relationship lasted only for about six months, because Brian—though he loved Esteban very much—wanted a life partner who was also a Jewish man.

What do you want in a man, spiritually? Do you want a guy who believes in a Higher Power? Is it important for you that a man belong to a particular denomination? Are you searching for a man who is your "karma buddy"? Do you want a man with whom you can have lengthy talks about spiritual matters? Do you have a desire to get married in a religious/spiritual ceremony? Do you want someone who is committed to social action in the context of a religious calling? Would you like to do Bible reading with someone? Are you interested in becoming a minister or rabbi, and so want someone who would support you in this calling?

Value-based

Values are the principles of life. What do you want in a man values-wise? Do you want a man who is principled regarding paying taxes and bills, and not fudging on financial matters? A man who has a deep commitment to protecting the environment? A man with a strong sense of ethics? A man who uses his power and influence to shape the political agenda? A man com-

mitted to fund-raising for the gay community? A man who volunteers his time for the community? A man committed to animal rights?

A gentleman I know, Giovanni, met his boyfriend at an AIDS
advocacy forum. His boyfriend is a political animal, fiercely committed to progressive causes. Giovanni found this passion both
sexy and infectious.

Sexual/Sensual

Now we've gotten to the good part! What do you want in a
man, sexually and sensually? Do you like a man who can sweep
you off your feet and take you places sexually you've never been
before? Do you want a man who is specifically a top or a bottom, a versatile man, or a man who is ambiguous and mysterious about what he does in bed, so that he can surprise you? Do
you want a man who talks dirty, talks sweetly, talks like he's in
charge, talks like *you're* in charge? Perhaps you want a man with
great hands, who can give you a sensual massage. This is a great
gift one man can give to another—healing and loving hands that
can soothe and relax. Are there some things you want sexually that you find hard to articulate? Do you like to wrestle with
your man, or perhaps give or receive a fun spanking? Do you
enjoy giving and/or receiving anal and/or oral sex? Remember: we're all different, and one's pleasure could be someone else's
turn-off.

What Preston, a workshop participant, wanted most in a
man sexually was an A+ kisser. Kissing was his acid test for a potential lover.

Cultural

What are your cultural priorities? Is it important for your future mate to share a cultural life with you? Do you want a man who appreciates fine art and museums, the theater, listening to a Bach cantata, relaxing to Mozart and white wine? What about a knowledge of specific musical styles: classical, rock, jazz, cabaret, Broadway musicals?

Desmond, a thirty-eight-year-old editor, is a culture vulture. He has five subscriptions to different cultural organizations, including the local symphony. Desmond started dating Martin, a twenty-nine-year-old investment banker who was more interested in reruns of *Friends.* Though Martin had other, wonderful qualities, Desmond found him to be "culturally deprived." So, without pushing his cultural tastes on Martin, Desmond would invite him along to various events.

"I bought tickets to *La Bohème,* and wasn't sure if Martin would go. He did, though, and was very moved by the opera, which surprised him, but not me. Martin didn't grow up with any exposure to culture, so I was kind of breaking him in. We now go to a lot of cultural stuff together. Martin even just bought a subscription series for us, to an experimental theater company which does some pretty edgy stuff. Though it's not my cup of tea, I'm glad to share this experience with Martin."

Specifics

Specific wants are crucial to some men; for others, they're less important. Some men who are short are not interested in tall men, and others could care less. For some men, the age of a man is an important factor in their choice; some personals ads might specify "I want a guy 28–35" or "36–45," but you will also see some that state "age unimportant." Do you like men with brown, blue, or green eyes? Is a specific weight range matched with height important? Do you want a man who is Italian, English, African American, Asian American, or Polish? Is a nonsmoking and/or vegetarian person important to you? There is nothing wrong with being specific, but understand that the more specific you are, the more limited the pool of available men who can match your specifications.

LET'S GET TO WORK

Part One: Sample Wants List

Have fun going through these 100+ wants, checking off those you find appealing. This list may stimulate your imagination, and prepare you for Part Two.

warm smile	likes dogs
mustache/facial hair	likes cats
sincere	open-minded
has own business	self-starter
physically fit	smoker
churchgoer	nonsmoker
confident	deep voice
likes to drive	enjoys family
enjoys money	likes sports
bald	likes outdoors
nice eyes	protective
hairy chest	great pecs
likes computers	soul mate

likes to eat out

a teddy bear

a big bear

sense of humor

nurturing

great cook

sensitive

loyal

likes his job

on a spiritual path

appreciates Eastern religions

likes to dance

thoughtful

intelligent

lives in the country

great kisser

bubble butt

walks with confidence

wild imagination

romantic

enjoys discussing current
events

does *Times* crossword

stable

not in debt

good listener

can balance checkbook

mature

makes a good salary

committed

good investments

enjoys dinner parties

good balance between
spending and saving
money

likes to go to clubs

likes to play cards with
friends

believes in Higher Power

enjoys having family over

likes to attend soccer games

meditates

chants

likes to smell me

enjoys films

likes ethnic food

full lips

has naughty side

good dresser

likes cuddling

self-possessed

good value-system

likes poetry

has good energy

wants children

a friend of Bill W.

into leather

enjoys nature

gives good massages

enjoys politics

likes to travel

buffed body

environmentally conscious

likes opera

independent nature

enjoys storytelling

career-oriented

supportive

likes the theater

enjoys espresso bars

voracious reader

speaks French

smooth body

creative

wears glasses

enjoys cocktails

city dweller

likes gardening

reads newspaper every day

spontaneous nature

homebody

Christian

Jewish

Muslim

agnostic

collects antiques

loyal

into animal rights

top

bottom

versatile

is gentle in bed

is an animal in bed

visits museums

enjoys Bach

enjoys Vivaldi

enjoys Mozart

age 35–46

of another race

vegetarian

Part Two: Choosing Your Wants

Now it's time to take out your pencil and paper, to choose which of your "wants" are most important to you. Put them into nine categories as listed above and on page 49. List as many wants as possible—a minimum of four per category. Find a comfortable and even meditative space to do this exercise in. *Don't rush.* Take as much time as you need. And don't edit yourself!

SAMPLE LIST (USE THIS FORMAT TO LIST *YOUR* WANTS)

INTELLECTUAL   voracious reader; speaks French; enjoys discussing current events; does *Times* crossword

EMOTIONAL   stable; loyal; good listener; mature; committed

SOCIAL   enjoys large dinner parties; likes to go to clubs; likes to play cards with friends; enjoys having family over; likes to attend soccer games

FINANCIAL   not in debt; can balance checkbook; makes a good salary; good investments; a good balance between spending and saving money

PHYSICAL   full lips; great pecs; mustache/facial hair; buffed body

SPIRITUAL   practices a specific religion (Mormonism, Catholicism, Judaism, Islam); has a spiritual path; believes in a Higher Power; meditates

VALUES   environmentalist; into animal rights; likes to volunteer; involved in community; member of school board

SEXUAL/SENSUAL   great kisser; top; gives great massages; is an animal in bed

CULTURAL   visits museums; likes opera; goes to the theater; enjoys foreign films; enjoys Bach/Vivaldi/Mozart

Part Three: Choosing Your Needs

After you list all of your wants, circle eight which are crucial to your choice of a mate. These will constitute your *needs*. You can choose these eight needs from any of the nine categories. For instance, if emotional needs are key to you, you may have three of those on your final "needs" list. If physical needs are important, choose one or more from that category. It all depends on you. Be truthful with yourself. This will be your starting point in choosing appropriate men to date.

Keep in mind *specific* needs that you may want to incorporate into your final needs list: nonsmoker, vegetarian, specific religion/race/age, etc.

Make note of the following as you winnow down your list:

- If you've been in a previous relationship, ask yourself which wants proved important, which did not, and which went unmet
- If you're new to the dating scene, ask yourself, "What would really make me happy and fulfilled with a guy?"
- "If I knew that I was going to grow old with this man, how would this affect my choices?"
- If you eliminate the word *should* from your choices—e.g., I *should* have a guy who looks like Brad Pitt, or the man *should* love classical music—what will your list look like?

After you complete your needs list, put it in some visible place in your home so that you always have a reminder of your highest priorities in choosing a man. Our needs can change over time—with experience, maturity, and insight—so you may want to review your list more than once.

Taking a Peek at Two Needs Lists

Peter's Needs

1. big bear
2. Christian
3. likes to travel
4. trusting
5. sense of humor
6. 35–50
7. is gainfully employed
8. HIV–

Why did Peter choose these eight needs?

Peter is a thirty-eight-year-old administrative assistant for a prestigious advertising agency. He makes $60,000+ a year. He is 5'11", 165 pounds, clean-cut, and he speaks Spanish and Portuguese. He's been in one five-year relationship, with a big bear, which ended amicably. Though conservative in appearance, Peter likes wild, burly men to snuggle up with in bed. One of the reasons his last relationship broke up was that his ex found it difficult to hold down a job and never had enough money—he had never really grown up. So Peter swore the next man he went out with had to be gainfully employed and satisfied with his work. He didn't have to earn a lot of money—just enough to be able to afford some of the pleasures of life. Peter now wants to travel, something he couldn't do with his ex, who could barely pay his rent.

Peter likes a guy with a naughty sense of humor and a big belly laugh—which his ex had. Peter goes to Metropolitan Community Church every Sunday and he requires that his prospective boyfriend be Christian. Peter has always been worried about HIV; though he knows his fear is a bit irrational and though he'd like to be more open, he needs an HIV− man. Race is unimportant to Peter. The person can smoke, but never in the house or car. Peter is also allergic to cats: no cat owners need apply.

I believe Peter's needs list is balanced and realistic. No "fantasy man" leaps out from the list. Peter is entering the dating world with a strong sense of who he is and what his needs are.

Langston's Needs
1. age 34−48
2. income $50,000+
3. likes long sensitive lovemaking
4. excellent shape—well built
5. progressive politics
6. understanding and kind
7. spiritual—no religions
8. likes films and the theater

Langston is a thirty-five-year-old African American, born in Baltimore, 5'10", 165 pounds, works in journalism, makes $50,000+ a year. Though he admits to being attracted to white men, Langston is open to all races. Langston came out when he was thirty-two and has dated only sporadically, but would like to settle down. Some of the men he has had sex with seem to rush and want to get it over with, so one of his needs is long, playful, soulful, and sensitive lovemaking. Though he's a top he'd be open to getting fucked by the right man—in a monogamous relationship. He grew up in a fundamentalist religion, so he shies away from men who are too religious. Langston wrote film reviews for his college paper and has great love for films and the stage; he'd like to share this love with a boyfriend. A guy doesn't have to be rich, but Langston would like to meet a guy who makes a good income and has opportunities for advancement.

Is it possible to have an unrealistic needs list? The answer is yes. William, thirty-two, had a seven-inch dick as a must on his list. I asked him if he would yield to a smaller penis and he said no. Another man, Jerome, said he absolutely needed a biker with tattoos and pierced nipples; Jerome would not negotiate this need. Dwight, a forty-eight-year-old retired investment banker, needed a man with a house in the country. For Lorenzo, a prospective mate had to be a born-again Christian.

If you find that you have included some nonnegotiable needs, such as those above, consider that this will decrease the number of men available to you. Make your needs list *realistic*. If you're fifty-three and are looking for a thirty-two-year-old with a hot body, you may (who knows?) win the dating lottery, but you may also be setting yourself up for failure.

A number of years ago I set a friend of mine up with a very handsome man who worked in television, was single, and had beautiful almond-shaped eyes. My friend agreed to meet him at a book-signing party. He called me that night and said, "He's handsome and really nice, but he has a fat butt." I almost died. I *never* thought the guy had a big butt, but my friend did. This man had every right to find the perfect-butt man, but I also believe he was limiting himself. He is still looking for a man with the perfect butt.

Kenneth, a sixty-year-old businessman, mature, distinguished, and handsome, told a friend he was looking to date another ma-

ture man: "No young guys—I don't have the energy." His needs
list included "mature man 55–70." Well, lo and behold, his
friend met someone at a yoga conference: a smart, good-looking
forty-four-year-old Asian man.

He introduced the younger man to Kenneth. The younger
man fell head over heels, and though Kenneth was quite flattered, he knew it would never work. *Much too young.* To make a
long story short, Kenneth, upon seeing other beautiful qualities
in the younger gentleman, agreed to date him. Kenneth was not
selling out on his needs as much as adjusting to some important
new information: that some younger people can be wise and mature, and that you can be flexible in allowing new people into
your life.

A good example of striking a balance is Topper, a forty-eight-
year-old actor who makes a good living doing voice-overs in a
small city. His needs list included: excellent shape; giver, not
taker; nice dick; good listener; makes $50,000+; nonsmoker;
sexually versatile; on a spiritual path.

Topper met a wonderful man who met all of the above needs
except one: nonsmoker. Lou kept the secret for a month. When
Topper heard that Lou smoked, he almost had a heart attack!
"Doesn't he know it could kill him? Why does he have to ruin
it?" On and on Topper went.

I asked Topper if there was any room for compromise with
Lou Camel, and he emphatically said no. "I have breathing dif-
ficulties, and I hate the smell, and I don't want to be around that
kind of pollution." So I asked Topper how much he liked Lou,
and he said a great deal. Then I asked him would he at least con-

sider talking to Lou about the smoking without issuing ultimatums, and he agreed to try.

After they spoke, Lou told Topper he would be willing to do the following: he would never smoke indoors, or in the car, or while dining. He would limit his cigarettes to three a day at most, and would make sure his clothes and mouth did not smell of smoke. And he would try never to smoke in front of Topper. So Topper said he was willing to give it a try. Topper and Lou have now been together for two years. For the first year, Topper didn't even realize that Lou smoked, except when they went on vacation and Lou would "go for a little walk." After a year, Lou stopped smoking. Topper ultimately engaged in a healthy compromise around his needs which, fortunately, were not written in stone.

You've had the opportunity in this chapter to take a good look at yourself, and to reflect on the person you are and want to be in the singles scene. Your needs list is the foundation for your work in the rest of this book and your future dating life. With your newfound knowledge and understanding, you are ready to learn the language of dating: what to say in approaching men for a date, and how to say it.

CHAPTER 2

BEGINNING THE CONVERSATION

A good line is hard to resist.

—MAE WEST, *KLONDIKE ANNIE*

Having completed the wants vs. needs exercise in the previous chapter, you have reaffirmed and reinforced your right to find a partner who will meet your most important needs. With this emotional foundation firmly in place, you are now prepared for the next step: learning and perfecting the art of casual conversation.

Are you a little awkward when you meet people, either casually, socially, or in dating situations? Do you hate making small talk and wince at using it? Actually, small talk can be quite fun once you get the skills down, and the payoff will be a social and love life you never thought possible. Put aside the prejudices you've developed due to glad-handing politicians and pesky salesmen. Small talk is socially useful. It makes networking possible and may open the way for a future romance. Everything you ever wanted to say to a man buy didn't know *how* to say is covered here.

LEVEL ONE: NEIGHBORHOOD SMALL TALK

This style of conversation keeps the world sane and friendly. Begin practicing small talk in your everyday life. It can be richly rewarding, and you'll find a remarkable change in the way you interact with your environment. Remember that being kind and friendly doesn't cost a cent. Developing a more positive attitude toward day-to-day connections will have a spillover effect in your dating life.

- "Beautiful day out today!"
- "We finally got this much-needed rain!"
- "How are your mom and dad doing?"
- "Do you have the time?"
- "Did the mail come yet?"
- "Great car!"

LEVEL TWO: SMALL TALK AT YOUR JOB

- "Great sweater!"
- "You look great! Were you on vacation?"
- "Nice tan!"
- "I saw a great movie, which I recommend!"
- "Have you seen the latest exhibition?"
- "Where have you been? We missed you!"

Note: practice small talk on a daily basis, so your casual conversation becomes as simple and easy as breathing.

LEVEL THREE: ICEBREAKERS FOR THE GAY-SINGLE LIFE

One of the most frequent questions I get from gay men is: What do I say to a man when I approach him? We all have so much anxious chatter in our heads, *anticipating* what we're going to say to a guy, that we're simply unaware of one simple, pleasant, and direct phrase that will open the gates of dating heaven . . .

> *While extending your right hand, say confidently, and with a big warm smile: "Hi, I'm Michael!"*

That's it. Many men have told me that the TWI—the three-word introduction—has jump-started very stimulating conversations. Now let's take some icebreakers and place them in the context of gay social situations.

Bookstore

You're browsing around a bookstore and suddenly make eye contact with this nice-looking guy in the fiction section. Your heart is thumping. "Oh, God, what do I say?" Take a deep breath and say, in a friendly manner: "Hi. I'm Steve. Can you recommend any good books?"

Neighborhood Park

You see Mr. Gorgeous sitting on a nearby bench. You want to go over and introduce yourself, but you hesitate, telling yourself, "I can't do that . . ." Don't *think* about it. You can! Approach your man with confidence and in your confident voice say: "Excuse me, I was sitting over there thinking of saying hello to you, but I was feeling kind of shy. So I decided—oh, what the heck! So I've come over to introduce myself. My name is John."

Believe me, this has worked! There are some very handsome guys out there who would love to receive the attention of a gentleman.

Community Social

You're at a local community meeting. There's a guy next to you who you know is gay. Smile, and gently say: "Hi. My name is Donnell. I don't know too much about this group. Have you been here before?"

Vestibule in Church/Synagogue

While you're waiting for the service to begin, you see an attractive man. Say: "Hi. I'm Javier. Do you attend services regularly?"

Supermarket

You're at the local supermarket. You see this guy who is ruggedly handsome and who looks familiar. A nice intro: "Excuse me, I'm sure I know you from somewhere, but I can't remember where. I'm Benjamin."

Gym

You're at the gym. It's a physical-fitness paradise, and you see this nice-looking guy ready to do some heavy lifting. You swagger over: "Need a spot?"

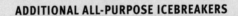

ADDITIONAL ALL-PURPOSE ICEBREAKERS

- Excuse me, I'm Carlos. I just want to tell you what beautiful eyes you have.
- That's a great leather jacket!
- Hi, I'm Paul. I just wanted to say that you have a marvelous smile.
- I'm new to this neighborhood. Do you know which are the good restaurants?
- I overheard you talking. You have a wild sense of humor!
- You have a great laugh.
- Weren't you in the marathon last year?
- I'm sorry for bothering you. May I borrow a pen?
- Great laptop. I'm looking to buy a new computer. Where did you get it?
- Excuse me, do you mind if I join you?
- I don't know anyone here. Do you?
- Hi, I'm Clark. You come here often?

Locker Room

You've seen this one guy a couple of times before, wearing a P-town T-shirt, but you've been too shy to approach him. Not anymore! Try: "I saw you working out upstairs. I just joined last week and wanted to introduce myself. I'm Frank."

Bar

You see a really cute guy and make some initial eye contact. Go over, extend your hand, give a friendly smile, and say: "Hi, I'm Clayton." That's the TWI. It works like a charm!

The vast majority of men will respond positively to an icebreaker. You may get a few attitude queens, but they are the exception to the rule. Icebreakers are just that—they get the social juices going. They help us to see if a guy is interested. Sometimes an icebreaker works, sometimes it doesn't. The trick is not to get hurt if it doesn't. When you get a positive response from an icebreaker, that's a win. And we need wins to keep up the momentum.

I told Clarence, one of my clients, about a singles night in Manhattan. He said he couldn't go by himself and he was unable to find a buddy who would go with him. I asked why he couldn't go alone. "It's too painful. I get this mini-agoraphobia, where everything becomes so vast and expansive, and I'm this little tiny dot at the singles event. Everyone else is a giant and I'm nobody." I worked with Clarence, telling him we would bookend the singles event: he could call me right before he left the house, as soon as he got to the event, and after he left. If I wasn't in, he could leave a message.

Clarence needed to feel that he was not alone as he was going through this process, and that whatever he decided to do was okay with me—though I'd be lying if I didn't admit I was rooting for him to attend the event! He did go, and—not to my surprise—had a very enjoyable time. The large room where the event was held was not that overwhelming, and the people running the event were extremely friendly. Clarence put on his name tag and met three different guys, two of whom gave him their number.

If you're not working with a therapist, make sure you have a friend you can call and speak with about your dating progress.

TEN OPEN-ENDED QUESTIONS THAT WORK

1. What brought you to (any geographical location: Los Angeles, Seattle, Atlanta)?
2. How did you get involved in (fund-raising, community theater, the stock market, producing)?
3. What was (any school: Stanford, Florida State, Williams) like?
4. What was it like growing up in (any city or geographical location: Cleveland, Europe, the South)?
5. Where did you learn how to (speak four languages, cook, kiss)?
6. What do you like about (Steven Spielberg, *Queer as Folk,* Hillary Clinton)?
7. What was (coming out, living in a small town, living in Las Vegas) like?
8. Tell me what it's like working for (Disney, the Stock Exchange, the *Los Angeles Times*)?
9. What do you like to do for fun?
10. What do you like to do on weekends?

LEVEL FOUR: CONTINUING THE CONVERSATION

Starting a conversation may be relatively easy compared to *continuing* the conversation. After they have used the icebreakers successfully, the question I get from many singles is: What do I say *next,* now that I've gotten the ball rolling?

I tell them to become active listeners. An active listener doesn't just *hear* what a guy says; he *listens,* with his heart and mind. He doesn't judge or try to fix the guy. (When you truly take in the other man, you keep those chattering monkeys at bay—the worry thoughts that will drain the life out of any conversation, thoughts like, "How am I doing?" "What does he think of me?" "Oh God, what do I say next?" "He must think I'm an idiot.")

Next, you use the technique of open-ended questions (for example, "What got you interested in politics?"). Open-ended questions invite a more thoughtful response than questions which can be answered in one word (like, "Do you enjoy classical music?"). I remember being on a first date with a gentleman who asked, "Who are your favorite writers?" I loved that question! And, of course, I gave an expansive answer.

LEVEL FIVE: PRE-DATES

Pre-dates are important. They are an invaluable way of "saying hello" to a man you met either online or through a personal ad. You can pick up a lot of information in a half hour. A pre-date is like a reconnaissance flight: you're checking him out to see if you want to go out on a regular date. Pre-dates are informal, spontaneous, and short. You can say, "Let's meet and introduce ourselves." The operative word is *introduction.* If he asks if this is a date, you can say, "I usually want to meet someone before I go on a date."

You may find the man you pre-date to be a fascinating future friend, but not a boyfriend. Or he may, indeed, be "boyfriend material," in which case you can get out your calendar and make a date. Or he may be someone with whom, for whatever reason, you don't want to spend more time.

Seamus is a thirty-six-year-old fashion designer who just came out of an eight-year relationship. Before getting hooked, Seamus was always being wooed and pursued by other guys. "I was really hot. Guys would come up to me and give me their

13 WAYS TO ASK A GUY OUT ON A PRE-DATE

(ALWAYS USE A FRIENDLY TONE OF VOICE AND *SMILE*.)

1. I had a nice time talking to you. Here's my number. Let's do coffee next week.
2. How's your schedule this week? I'd like to meet you for tea and talk some more.
3. I'm a big fan of yours. I'm working on a special project, and was wondering if you'd like to join me at Starbucks for a quick coffee.
4. I'm Pete. I believe we're in the same bowling league. I've been wanting to ask someone about the finals tournament. Do you have time for coffee?
5. Congratulations on your promotion! I'd like to take you out for a drink.
6. I'm Fernando. I think we go to the same laundry. I'm the greedy one who takes up three machines. Would you like to grab a cappuccino?
7. Hi! Didn't I see you at the city planning board meeting last month? I'm George. I like what you said about the dog ordinance. I'm headed for a drink. Interested in joining me?
8. I love your cabaret work. I saw your performance last week. I'd like to take you out for a drink to celebrate your opening.
9. I think we belong to the same gym. I've seen you working out and been wanting to say hello for a while. I'm Sebastian. I'm headed to get a smoothie. Care to join me?
10. I'm Dennis. I've been coming to this fellowship for a while. I'm trying to make some contacts. Do you want to get some tea?
11. Hi. I'm Nelson. I'm new to this law firm. I'd like to ask you to join me for coffee in the cafeteria.
12. You're a great dancer. You belong on Broadway! I'd like to buy you a drink. I'm Pedro.
13. Didn't you work at Crown publishing last year? Hi, I'm Leonard; I'm a literary agent. I thought you looked familiar! I'm headed for coffee. Want to join me?

number for no reason. Now that I'm single again, the bloom is off the rose. It hasn't been easy. I've actually become really shy." Seamus—a sweet guy who likes to be everybody's friend, but who sometimes forgets to take care of himself—couldn't even ask a guy out for coffee. I told him that men love guys with confidence, guys who take the initiative and go after what they want.

I asked Seamus to set a goal of getting six pre-dates over the period of a month. I thought he would collapse in my office! "Six pre-dates! How about one!" I knew he could do it, but he had major doubts. So we went over a list of pre-date phrases, improvising our way through a session.

LEVEL SIX: DATE-DATE

The date-date is when you ask out a man you are interested in on a real, honest-to-God date. You might not use the word *date*, but—unless he's a little dull—he'll know and be flattered. (You may, also, ask a man for his card and e-mail him to ask him out.) But before you ask someone out, make sure he's single! Ask: "Are you single?" "Do you have a boyfriend?" "Are you in a relationship?"

When you ask a man out for a date-date, don't go to each other's home either before or after. There is too much temptation to have sex or to be thinking about sex in such a setting, and first dates are about getting to know someone, not going all the way. Stay in neutral territory!

12 SIMPLE, DIRECT WAYS TO ASK
A GUY OUT FOR A DATE

1. I'd like to go out on a date with you.
2. Are you interested in dinner on Friday night?
3. I'd really like to get to know you better. Are you available for brunch this weekend?
4. This is hard for me, but I've been wanting to ask you out for a month.
5. I see you every day and never get a chance to talk to you. What are you doing on Friday night?
6. Hey, wanna go out on a date?
7. What are you doing on Saturday night?
8. I'm not good at this, but I think you're a cool guy and I want to ask you out.
9. My astrologer said I should ask out a Gemini. What are you doing this weekend?
10. I have two tickets for the theater on Saturday afternoon. Are you interested in joining me?
11. I hardly know you, but I'd like to ask you out for a drink.
12. You're a good-looking guy, and I'm not going to beat around the bush. Are you interested in joining me for dinner Saturday night?

DATING AND THE RIPPLE EFFECT

At times the dating scene appears incredibly overwhelming. Where do I start? Where do I meet guys? I tell many men to just start the ball rolling by extending their social network and creating a "ripple effect." A ripple effect is an unintended effect: the more action we take, the greater the ripple effect. For example, if I go to the Metropolitan Community Church and join their men's support group, I have now come into contact with twenty-five to seventy-five men on the spot. As I get to know people and develop friendships, I'm going to be invited to parties and get-togethers by fellow congregants. At these parties, there's an excellent chance I'll meet other singles whom I can invite to my annual Christmas brunch. Then, I'll be invited to another man's Valentine's party. With the ripple effect, the possibilities are endless.

Here are four success stories of men who took action and created their own ripple effects. Each threw his pebble into the dating waters and produced some wonderful, unintentional ripples.

The Hiking Club—Minneapolis

Adam was never a joiner. He'd go to different bars and occasionally attend a lecture at the gay center. Otherwise, he had two close friends: a woman who lived next door and a man he met at work. Every Sunday, he and his neighbor had a standing date for brunch.

Adam's social life had become comfortable and predictable, so he wanted to move outside his comfort zone. Then he saw a blurb in the local paper for a hiking club. Adam, who has hiked for years—mostly alone—finally got up the nerve to investigate joining a club. He wanted to share those "peak experiences" (witnessing a beautiful stream, purple-hued mountains, a rare bird species) while hiking with others. He called the group leader and arranged to meet for the next hike at a state park. Though the group was mostly straight, his "gaydar" sent him walking beside George, an attractive older man with a closely cropped beard.

George said, "There was this fabulous sunset last week," which tipped Adam off that George might be gay. They spoke in generalities, and then Adam said that he has a friend who works with people with HIV, and George told him that he does volunteer massage work at the local AIDS support organization. Adam had found a wonderful hiking companion!

George told Adam about a rafting trip he had been on with a gay group, and this inspired Adam to call them and get the info. "If George can do river rafting, so can I!" He made arrangements to go rafting with the group as well as to hike down the Grand Canyon.

When Adam got back to Minneapolis, he and George started a gay hiking club. Adam would never have thought, in a million years, that his social life would become so active. As he looks back, he realizes that some of his "craving for solitude" was mostly a form of isolation and fear of the unknown. He still likes his solitude, but in moderation only. He had no idea of the variety of riches within the gay community.

The Local Church—New Jersey

Matt, a twenty-five-year-old teacher, grew up in southern New Jersey and attended Rutgers University, where he came out at age nineteen. Though he was a member of three clubs as an undergraduate, Matt's social life after school was nil. His idea of a date was ordering Chinese food and watching *Sex and the City*—alone. He was in a rut and didn't even know it. To break the monotony, he would rent some porn or call a phone-sex line.

One Sunday, Matt noticed an announcement in his church bulletin for a gay social-action group that met once a week. Matt had always been shy, and the notion of going to this meeting made him a little anxious. The usual negative thoughts raced through his head: "No one will be there"; "What do I say when I arrive?" But all of a sudden, something clicked in his brain. He remembered what his minister had said about doing service and helping out in the community, and this impressed him very much. There was a contact name and number in the bulletin for the social-action group, so Matt called and introduced himself. The coordinator, Carlos, told Matt that about fifteen people usually showed up at the meetings, and he would be most welcome.

Though a little scared, Matt said to himself, "Fuck it," and made a commitment to show up on Monday. The agenda for that evening was to organize a bus ride to Washington, D.C., for an anti-violence rally. Matt volunteered to put together a flyer for the event.

The bus ride to D.C. forced Matt to confront his shyness. He was worried at first: "Who will sit next to me on the way down to Washington?" "What am I going to say?" "Am I going to feel stuck—trapped—the whole trip?" As he walked onto the bus, there were only about six empty seats, so he gathered his courage and sat down next to a man named Craig, who had been a member of the church for twelve years. The conversation went much more smoothly than Matt could ever have expected. In fact, Matt found himself talking too much!

Over the next six months, Matt worked together with Craig on a number of projects, including setting up a food pantry for the homeless. They became close friends. Social events at the church became less threatening as Matt developed a network of friends. He always looked forward to the monthly potluck supper sponsored by the gay men's church fellowship, and he joined the local gay chorus.

Matt had finally found the affiliation he was always looking for. For the first time in five years, he started dating. The confidence that Matt developed from interacting with church members was spilling over to his personal life. The ripple effect was in full force.

Acting Class—New York City

Tom is an actor and very much in the closet. Though Tom has a close network of friends (mostly straight), he has always kept a distance from the gay community. As Tom pursued his acting career with feverish intensity, he knew there was something missing in his life. He wanted to fall in love. Looking back, he says it was after his thirty-fifth-birthday party that the idea of "getting older" hit him like a sledgehammer.

One day, a gay friend told him about and invited him to "Queer Stories," a group of gay men that met at the LGBT Center every Saturday to tell their own stories about growing up gay. Some men prepared their stories beforehand, others got up and performed spontaneously. The thought of going to such a gathering panicked Tom. Along with everything else, the LGBT Center was off-limits: if he was seen there, it would be guilt by association. He politely declined his friend's offer.

A couple of months later, Tom's friend called him again with the same invitation. Tom hesitantly said yes. When he got to the large room where "Queer Stories" met, he immediately went to the back of the room while his friend took a seat up front.

Tom watched and watched, and became mesmerized by the performances. At the end of the event, Tom joined the group for lunch, and was so moved by the infectious enthusiasm and camaraderie of the men that he agreed to give it a whirl—to perform the following Saturday.

The next week, Tom told about growing up gay outside Milwaukee, and how he loved, as a fourteen-year-old, watching his twentysomething neighbor, Warren, mow the lawn on Saturday mornings, shirtless. He spoke about his crushes, his disappointments, and the fear of being "caught being gay" by guys on the soccer team. He got through the performance without a hitch, and received wild applause.

One day on his way up to the room for "Queer Stories," Tom stopped off at the large community bulletin board to check out the flyers. He locked eyes with a great-looking man and, on impulse, introduced himself. "Hi. I'm Tom," he said. "Oh, I'm Nick," the other man answered. Tom told Nick about "Queer Stories," and Nick said he would like to go sometime, but had other business that day. Tom gave Nick his telephone number and told him to call when he decided to come. Nick didn't wait till then. He called Tom the next day, and later that week they went on a very successful first date.

Tom's story is not unique. By showing up for himself, he was able to overcome a lot of the baggage of internalized homophobia. Though scared at times, he continues to take actions that bring joy to his life.

Volunteer Work—Boston

Joseph, forty-three, works as a successful creative director at an advertising agency in Boston. Joseph was married to a woman for five years and came out when he was thirty-five. He's had a series of boyfriends, the longest lasting four months. Joseph hadn't dated anyone for two years.

He ran a personal in the local gay newspaper and got thirty responses, but only responded to two, which resulted in one-night stands. He came home from work exhausted each night, and on weekends went grocery shopping, did the laundry, and headed to the gym. Except for an occasional discreet blowjob at the gym, his sex, social, and romantic life was zilch. He thought everyone at the gym was an "attitude queen," including himself.

On his way home from work one night, Joseph was struck by a poster seeking volunteers for a new gay community theater. Intrigued, he called, and Rose, the theater's director, gave him a quick history of the company, which was embarking upon a major fund-raising effort and needed a person who could "sell" the theater concept to potential donors. Rose told Joseph his help would be enormously appreciated.

Joseph began working at least ten hours a week at the theater, and loved every moment. The staff and actors could not have been nicer. After two months, he helped them launch what was to become an extremely successful fund-raising drive.

Rose and her partner, Alexandria, had bi-weekly potluck suppers at their home, where Joseph got to know a whole new group of queer men and women. In a short period of time, he had extended his social network beyond his wildest dreams. On weekends—during which, in the past, he might have received one or two calls from friends—he now would get six or seven calls. He felt alive again, and life began to feel worth living.

At a volunteers' barbecue on Memorial Day Joseph met Howard, a teacher in a Boston public high school. They hit it off, and dated for a month before deciding to spend a weekend together in Provincetown. The concept of a soul mate was an abstraction for Joseph until he met Howard. For the first time in his life, he knew what it meant to belong to someone.

All of the men in these stories demonstrate how the ripple effect can produce very positive results in the social and dating life of even the most resistant, doubt-ridden man. Sometimes the tiniest action can produce astounding results, so think small at first. What is that one action you can take that jump-starts your social and love life? Is it volunteering? Is it joining a hikers' club? Is it coming out? (Not so small!) Is it joining a group at your local church?

Remember: there are men out there dying to meet you. Get going!

SOCIAL ACTIVITIES FOR GAY MEN

Local Health Club/Gym

Check out special lecture-presentations on nutrition, body fat, stress reduction, acupuncture, safer sex. Make sure you say hello to the man sitting next to you.

Spiritual Groups

Most organized religions and queer spirituality groups have fellowship meetings, potlucks, and socials. You *don't* have to be a member to show up for most gatherings. Gay spiritual groups are amazingly hospitable. There's a home waiting for you.

Parties/Holidays/Events

Check your local gay newspaper for upcoming activities. It's shocking how many men don't read the local gay-events listings. If gay Greeks are having their Christmas party, check with the coordinator to see if you can show up—even if you're not Greek. If queer bankers are having an "Evening Under the Stars," find out if it's an open event and attend, even if you're an English teacher.

Gay Sports/Outdoors and Social Clubs

You name the club and there will be gay singles there.

Sports clubs
- Scuba Diving
- 4-Wheel Drive
- Ski
- Motorcycle
- Bikers
- Bowling
- Hiking
- Running
- Yachting
- Rodeo
- Wrestling
- Martial Arts
- Snowboarding
- Tennis
- Hockey
- Softball
- Aquatics
- Basketball
- Baseball
- Soccer
- Gay Games
- Football
- Mountain Climbing
- Equestrian . . .

Special interest
- Imperial Court
- S/M
- Gay Fathers
- Girth and Mirth
- Student Unions
- Naturists/Nudists
- Reading Groups
- Vintage Cars
- Twentysomething
- Thirtysomething
- Gardening

Camping
Cheerleading
Leather/Levi's
Bears
Ballroom Dancing
Amateur Radio
Square Dancing . . .

Gay professional organizations
Physicians
Lawyers
Teachers
Architects
Police Officers
Bankers

Publishers
People in Fashion
Dentists
Psychiatrists
Psychotherapists . . .

Ethnic groups
African American
Asian
Italian
Mexican
Polish
Greek
Latino
German . . .

Remember: there are many other groups to consider. And if there's a specific group you want to join that doesn't exist in your area, start it yourself!

CRUISING VS. FLIRTING

The ripple effect showed us how to get into the dating loop. Adam, Matt, Tom, and Joseph put themselves out there and were able to connect with organizations and people that would bring them community and the love they'd always been looking for. Their stories attest to the courage it takes for every man to move beyond the limitations of his comfort zone—and the rewards of doing so.

Moving from cruising to flirting, for many gay men, will be

CRUISING VS. FLIRTING

Cruising is retro	Flirting is post-gay
Cruising is getting a quickie	Flirting is take-your-time
Cruising is genitally focused	Flirting takes in the whole man
Cruising, you go to a guy's house to fuck	Flirting, you go to a guy's house to watch *Queer as Folk*
Cruising is intense focus of eyes	Flirting is soft focus of eyes
Cruising, you grunt	Flirting, you engage in casual conversation
Cruising, you carry condoms	Flirting, you carry a rose
Cruising, you have a hard look	Flirting, you smile
Cruising results in sex	Flirting results in dating
Cruising, you keep emotional distance	Flirting, you're approachable
Cruising, you grab each other's crotch	Flirting, you shake hands
Cruising, you don't care what you wear	Flirting is always neat/casual
Cruising has a dark and dangerous vibe	Flirting has a more open and fun vibe

a challenge. Cruising is so embedded in the culture of gay life that the very idea of questioning its value will raise some hackles. I assure you, I am not proposing to kill off cruising as much as to provide an alternative: *flirting*.

Danny is a twenty-nine-year-old political consultant with "dark Irish" good looks. He's a charmer who talks a mile a minute. Danny called me for a consultation and said, "I was always a good cruiser. I have intense eyes that could get guys in bed in ten minutes. I don't know how to be sexy without fucking. I want to be *romantic*. I'm approaching thirty—getting too old—and it scares me." He continued, "I have this romantic fantasy about sweeping this hot, nerdy guy off his feet." Danny also said he was tired of using recreational drugs, of late nights, and of "serial playmates."

"So you want to learn how to flirt?" I asked him. Danny looked puzzled. "Isn't flirting the same as cruising and cock-teasing?" I told him that men who cruise are playing games; flirting men are into romance, and want to attract and woo a man for dating, courtship, and a long-term relationship. I told Danny that cruising is not bad for getting laid, but is a dead end for relationship-minded guys. Flirting requires more specific skills.

Danny is not the only gay man alive who is confused about cruising and flirting. The short and simple definition of cruising is making the rounds to have sex. Cruising is giving off "I'm ready to fuck" vibrations. Flirting has a little more nuance to it. It is a relaxing, casual, and, most of all, charming way of getting a guy's attention without going all the way. It's about giving off "I'm ready for romance" vibrations.

Flirters need to be curious about other people—you become a flirting detective. When you're in a gay environment (social event/bar/coffee shop) take in, visually and auditorily, all the men around you. Notice everything about them, and you'll discover incredible diversity in the gay community. An acting teacher may encourage you to sit in parks, cafés, or on front porches to observe people. I want you to do the same. For instance, watch how men walk, how they carry themselves. Do they have a heavy walk, like they're carrying the weight of the world on their shoulders? Do they have a lively and carefree gait, as if the world is their oyster?

There's a difference between just *looking* at people and *taking them in.* When you take people in, you look at their eyebrows, rings, hair, tattoos, nose, goatee, legs, how they move their hands, how they talk, how they laugh. You find out what's unique, specific, and even peculiar about each person. You can gather so much information about people purely through the joys of observation!

The Hunt Begins—Danny's Story (continued)

Danny decided to visit a popular café in his predominantly gay neighborhood. "I see a man who looks quite interesting in a café. He's wearing a beret—and I usually hate berets—but this man wears it well. I notice that he orders cappuccino and lifts the cup with a certain grace. He's reading what look likes a travel book. I wonder where he's going. I watch some more, and this man starts to look very interesting. I page through last month's *People* magazine, peeking over at his every move and running mental statistics: 6'1", late thirties, 190 pounds. Then—uh-oh! Those monkeys start chattering in my head: 'Oh, forget about it, silly fool. He's probably waiting for his husband so they can trot off to couple's counseling.' Or: 'Oh no. I'll bet he's spending some time here before he catches the next movie. I won't have time to make my move.'

"He's looking more attractive by the moment, and if I let this opportunity go by without at least smiling or winking at him, I will forever be a sissy dater! So I go up to get another caramel frappuccino. As I move back toward my table, I stop by this guy and say, 'I'm sorry for bothering you, but I noticed your travel book and I'm looking to buy some new travel books.' (Liar!) 'Do you have any suggestions?' The man with the beret gives me this beautiful smile and says, 'Oh, sure. This is *Fodor's*—it's a great book. Where are you traveling to?' Quick—second lie: 'Oh, someplace in the Caribbean, with great cabana boys!' Oh no! Stupid. Stupid. Stupid. He laughs and says, 'I've been to Puerto Rico and St. Thomas and love them both. I can recommend a few places.' 'Oh, that would be great.' And then, with great aplomb, he asks, 'Why don't you join me?' Flustered, I say, 'Oh, I don't want to disturb you.' 'Not at all—I could use some company.' So we talk, and then I have to go (the truth!) to meet my friend. This man's name is Frank, and we exchange numbers. I call him the next day and ask if he's interested in joining me for dinner on Friday night. He agrees. I also ask him if he's single. He says yes."

Danny did a great job at the café. I'd give him an A+. He took in the man he was observing with great detail. There was a special vibe he picked up from Frank, and he pursued a very advanced course of action: going up to a man and introducing himself with an icebreaker. Notice he got flustered because Frank was so nice (yes, they're out there, guys!) but he kept his cool and stayed on course. Remember: Danny could cruise and fuck, but flirting was a totally new way of interacting for him. Danny was on the road to becoming a "Master Flirter."

Flirting needs to be fun and spontaneous. Though Danny had the ordinary jitters about going up to a man, he kept a sense of humor through the interchange. While you're doing the dating field-trip exercise below, keep your humor and relax.

Here is a list of tips for you to consider when you go into a café or other gay milieu. While in school, some of you went on field trips to the museum, the apple orchard, the mayor's office, the zoo. Well, this may be your first all-gay field trip to a gay café.

Flirting Field Trip

- Wear clothes you feel comfortable and sexy in.
- Walk into the café with confidence.
- Smile as you're surveying the room with soft-focused eyes.
- No attitude.
- Buy a refreshment.
- Take a seat where you can see and flirt with other guys—location is everything.
- Do something: read a book, magazine, newspaper, bring a laptop—these are your props; don't cover your face with the newspaper.
- Pick up cues/vibes.
- If a guy looks over at you, smile back—nothing more to do.
- Choose one person to use an icebreaker with: "Do you have the time?" "Interesting book you're reading." "Excuse me, have you been here before?" "I've never been here before . . ."

Or use other lines that allude to your shyness. They are often good starters, because they make you less threatening.

- If things are cooking, you can take the conversation to another level—beyond small talk—to something slightly personal. But pay attention to nonverbal cues! Is his body posture open to you, or has he withdrawn or turned away during the conversation?
- Answer rejection with a four letter word: "Next!"
- No cruising or picking up guys.

Two don'ts

- Don't have dishonest intentions. You are flirting. Be honest with yourself about what you *really* want from the interaction.
- Remember: no zingers. If you meet a guy in a bar, don't ask, "Do you come here a *lot*?" implying he's a barfly. Avoid approaching with a barb (e.g., "Hey, I haven't seen you at the gym in a long time. Taking it easy, eh?").

The exercise above can be risky for some men. It is not easy to put yourself out there and face the possibility of rejection. Meeting new people is real "grown-up" work, and requires a certain mental and emotional stamina. It will bring up an array of feelings: bashful, shy, nervous, terrified, abandoned—as well as tender, delighted, hopeful, silly, kind, and erotic.

Honor every feeling that comes up, without judgment. Don't beat yourself to a pulp mercilessly. Have "tender mercy" on yourself. Talk to people about your dating: friends, a therapist, a support group. *Never* feel like you're alone on this journey. It's always better to have someone at your side, gently nudging you along and saying, "You're doing great. Nothing ventured, nothing gained."

DATING FOR THE SUCCESSFUL MAN

The art of flirting is an advanced course in verbal and nonverbal communication which will bring you closer to your goal of approaching and being approached by others. It "screams" risky, but has a big payoff: getting great guys to meet. If you can flirt, you can date.

Are you one of the thousands of successful men who are highly talented in their careers and professional life, but just can't seem to get your love life together? Brad is a thirty-five-year-old investment banker who travels three months a year. He grew up in Massachusetts and went to Brown. He now lives in Boston. "I have everything but a mate. People always tell me I'm a great catch, that I'm 'boyfriend material.' I used to take that as a compliment. Now it just depresses me."

A self-admitted workaholic, Brad puts in sixty-hour weeks, works on weekends, and makes and receives business calls at home. "I can't seem to stop working. I love my job, but it takes its toll. I see my life passing by. I have more than enough money to live comfortably. My big secret is that escorts are my love life."

Brad fell in love with one of his escorts, Freddy, a twenty-one-year-old college kid from Vancouver. Brad took Freddy to South Beach, and when he looked at photos of the trip, it startled him to realize how young Freddy looked next to him. "My God, he was like a puppy! It was a wake-up call. I vowed never to use escorts again. It broke my heart."

Ripe for a relationship, Brad grieved the loss of Freddy, but knew that it was time to move on and get a romantic life. I worked on *time prioritizing* with Brad. First, I asked him, "Do you want to meet someone?" "Yes," he replied. Then I told him he was going to have to change his work schedule in order to make time for dating; otherwise, I could not work with him. He'd only be wasting his time and money.

I told Brad the key was to balance work with pleasure. I gave him the following categories and told him to fill in the approximate percentage of his time that he gave to each. The percentage should add up to a total of 100%.

Brad—old allocation of time

Career	70%
Volunteer work	0%
Dating	0%
Hobbies	2%
Friends and Family	5%
Recreation and Culture	5%
Spirituality	1%
Self-care (massages, facials)	0%
Gym	5%
Chores	10%
Other not listed (therapy, medical)	2%

When Brad looked at his allocation numbers, they stunned him. I asked him to write down new percentages for his future allocation of time, by the following week, and he became resistant. He thought of time as an enemy. I told him that time must be his friend or he will live the old life of Scrooge—all work and no fun.

Brad came back in two weeks with the following breakdown of time:

Brad—new allocation of time

Career	57%
Volunteer work	1%
Dating	5%
Hobbies	2%
Friends and Family	7%
Recreation and Culture	7%
Spirituality	2%
Self-care	2%
Gym	5%
Chores	10%
Other	2%

How was he going to accomplish this? He decided he would not work on weekends and would not take business calls at home in the evening. He would tell his boss that he had personal commitments to take care of and needed to cut back on business travel. He knew that his income might take a slight dip, but he was willing to do this for the sake of his sanity—and to bring more joy into his life.

Transferable Skills

Brad was able to use his business-world organizational skills to reorganize his personal life. He was transferring his skills.

Lots of professional men look almost hopeless when they come to me. But as soon as we engage the concept of transferable skills and put it into action, their dating takes on a life of its own.

Transferable skill #1: networking

Darren, thirty-four, has a high position at IBM, in which people skills are key. His job requires a lot of networking—meeting people from different divisions within IBM and making sure everyone's happy. Though Darren is quite pleasant to the eye, there is a shy side to him that has kept his dating life on hold. When he told me about his work at IBM, I said to Darren, "You have wonderful people skills. People naturally like you. *I* like you. You have a lot to offer. You're a little shy, because dating is risky. You're going to have to move out of the comfort zone of corporate IBM."

Darrren was a get-up-and-go person, so I suggested he join two organizations over the next month. (He told me he works better within groups/organizations than by going to bars.) He chose Frontrunners and a gay soccer team. Part of his dating action plan was to meet three new people from both the running club and the soccer team. He would introduce himself with a smile, shaking hands and saying, "Hi, I'm Darren." Just as he's done a thousand times at IBM!

Transferable skill #2: listening

Herman, forty, is a counselor at a local hospital. Over time, he has developed an extraordinary ability to listen to his clients. Herman came to me a little humbled: now *he* was sitting in the client's chair! Herman has rough good looks, is very smart, and has a sensitivity that would make anyone in his presence feel very welcome.

Herman came to me after his partner of fourteen years died of complications from AIDS. He found the singles scene very daunting and didn't know where to start. "I can't fathom going to a bar. When I think of other places, like the gay community center, it seems a bit overwhelming. This is all new to me. I'm not even sure what to say to guys on dates."

I told Herman that he comes across as a charming man, and that he would be just fine if he listened to the men that he met, picking up their cues and using the soft gaze of his eyes while looking at them. He's not "playing therapist"; he's using his professional skills of listening and being attentive—in the dating world. He already has the capacity to see the real, live human beings before him—a skill unfortunately lacking among some beginning daters.

Transferable skill #3: taking risks

If you want to increase your success, double your failure rate.

—THOMAS WATSON, FOUNDER OF IBM

Anton had a successful small business designing T-shirts for girls ages 9–14. Over the last five years, he's probably taken more than a dozen major risks involving his business. "There's never a dull moment, and it drives me crazy at times, but I love my business. It's like my child."

Anton wanted to meet guys, but he got quite lazy about it. "My only dates have been with my right hand. It's cheap, but not getting me anywhere. I keep putting dating on the back burner, and I know from my own business that if I don't do anything, nothing will get done."

I told Anton that I admired him for his business acumen and the risks he takes every day. "Owning a business requires risks," I said. "Now I want you to incorporate risks into your dating life." Gay Pride Week was coming up, and I gave Anton the challenge of getting ten names and telephone numbers from single guys, and of getting three dates from among those ten. No sex—dates only.

Anton was game, and up to the challenge. Not only did he get ten names, but he met a guy at the big outdoor dance and started dating him. When he came to see me two weeks later, he had been on four dates!

Tips for the Professional Man Who Has Everything but Love

- If someone asks you about your previous relationships and you haven't had any, you can say: "I've been working very hard at my career and have been pretty successful. That's the good news. The bad news is I've put my love life on the back burner, and haven't been doing a lot of dating."
- Workaholism is acceptable in our society. But it is a disease that can have dire consequences, not the least being the loss of happiness in one's life. If you're a workaholic, watch the film *Dead Poets Society* as an object lesson in the transitory nature of life.
- Don't take dating so seriously! Be humble. No divas need apply! Leave your corporate logo and ego at the office. And please, have a sense of humor—it's part of your gay gene pool!
- You need a win. A win has immediacy and will provide you

with more motivation. A win may be as simple as going up
to a man at a gay event and introducing yourself. Stay out of
your head ("Oh, what if he doesn't like me?"). Just do it!

- If a man rejects you, it may hurt, but don't take it personally.
Rejection is only a two-letter word: "no." Move on! Dwelling
on rejection will only make you angry and depressed, and
will take the fun and joy out of dating.

- Having the right mind-set is crucial to healthy dating. When
we're focused and centered, there is much less chance for
negative attitudes to set in.

- Show your confidence. Men love confident guys! If you feel
confident in your work life, but not in dating situations, act
"as if." You may not *feel* confident dating, but you can fake it
until you make it!

- Be accountable. Consider this a dater's "Weight Watchers":
you need to know how you're doing and what progress you've
made. Say, "I plan to get two dates within a week," and then
do it!

GETTING A DATE IN ONE MINUTE FLAT

Serendipity, risk, and spontaneity are the three ingredients in
getting a date in one minute flat. Serendipity is "the phenomenon of finding valuable or agreeable things not sought for." Risk
is taking a chance without thinking of the outcome. And spontaneity is "acting from a momentary impulse."

I frequently tell clients that it's possible to get a date in one
minute flat. Some men don't believe me, particularly those who
haven't dated for a long time and can't conceive how it can be

arranged in so short a time. So I tell them how *I* got a date in one minute flat—on the subway.

I was taking the uptown no. 1 train to Lincoln Center. It was on a Sunday, around one in the afternoon. As the train was approaching Sixty-sixth Street, I noticed a handsome African American man looking at me, and I looked back at him, and we both smiled. As I started to get off, I looked back, and he was still looking at me. As the doors were just ready to close, the gentleman got off the train and walked toward me.

EDMOND: Hi. I'm heading to Ninety-sixth Street, but I thought I'd say hello.

JIM: Glad you did. I'm Jim. [*shaking hands*]

EDMOND: I'm Edmond. What's up? Where are you off to?

JIM: I'm meeting a friend, and we're going to see *The Nutcracker.* How about you?

EDMOND: I'm going home. I was doing some shopping downtown and bought some new clothes.

JIM: I'm glad I met you, but I've got to run and meet my friend. Let me give you my number. I hope we can continue the conversation.

EDMOND: I'll give you mine also.

JIM: Great. I'll give you a call.

EDMOND: Sounds good. I'd like to know how *The Nutcracker* is.

JIM: Okay. I'll call you.

Edmond and I had a few nice dates. I believe there was an element of serendipity in our meeting. Edmond certainly took a risk, and the spontaneity of the moment took over.

The One-Minute Encounter

The theater, Friday night, Hairspray *intermission*

JAIME: Enjoying the show?

MARC: Yeah, it's great; especially the lead!

JAIME: The whole cast is great!

MARC: I'm a theater buff. I go to everything. I was really looking forward to this.

JAIME: So was I. This is my third play this month!

MARC: You're kidding! You beat me. This is my second show.

JAIME: What did you see?

MARC: *Oklahoma!* It was fantastic.

JAIME: Yeah, I saw it. Loved it. [*extends hand and smiles*] Hi. I'm Jaime. It's good to meet you.

MARC: I'm Marc. Good to meet you!

JAIME: [*hears theater bell*] I gotta go to my seat. Hey, what are you doing after the show? Would you like to join me for coffee and give your review?

MARC: Sure. That would be fun. How about we meet under the marquee?

JAIME: You got it! See you outside. Enjoy the second act!

MARC: Thanks. See you later!

CHAPTER 3

WHERE TO MEET GUYS

As you approach your dating life, remember: *spaces in which to meet available men are no longer confined to gay bars/clubs. One can meet an available man anywhere, anytime.*

So, think big; think smart; think new.

THINK BIG

Never limit yourself when you think about places to meet men. Joseph, thirty-four, said he was going to the Gay Games and, by the end of the games, he would find himself a boyfriend—and he did. He had to invest some money in this "Boyfriend Hunt," but it paid off. Joseph had challenged his old belief, that "there are no good places to meet singles."

Singles should use their ingenuity to generate their own lists of creative places to meet guys.

THINK SMART

What kind of guys do you want to meet? You may meet single guys at two A.M. on a Saturday night at your local watering hole, but is that the best place to find guys who are emotionally available? God gave you a brain: use it!

Going to a couple of Gay Pride marches in different cities might pay off. Many cities have an annual gay/lesbian film festival: find out if there is an opening-night cocktail party; ask if they need any volunteers—you can get in free and have the opportunity to work with fellow film lovers, shoulder to shoulder.

THINK NEW

You may think meeting singles at the gay rodeo is ridiculous, but how do you know there isn't some hunk there, ready to lasso you to his side? If they're having a "Big Bear" beauty contest at the local bar, why not enter the contest yourself (if you're a bear) or attend the event (even if you're not the perfect bear)? You can bet there'll be single bears waiting to meet you.

Have you ever entered a drag show, or at least gone to one? Show up, have some fun, and meet other men!

DATING AND THE NET

There is a deep human desire to connect, and the Internet helps fulfill this desire in breathtaking proportions. If I'm living in Minneapolis and want to connect with a Latino Londoner, I can do so in a very short period of time. The Internet is more than quick—it's instantaneous. For shy guys and men coming out, the Net is an enormous gift. Bashful guys can open up to other men online as they never would in real life. They can keep their shyness at bay; or, if they tell people they're shy, they needn't suffer the self-consciousness that might occur in a face-to-face meeting. Shy men can practice their communication skills and open up emotionally on the Net, without being overwhelmed by the fear of rejection.

The Net can be a singles Disneyland for the coming-out man, whether he's eighteen or over fifty. He can explore all aspects of the gay culture, from gay bankers, marathon runners, teachers, and musicians to drag queens, S/M activists, spiritual seekers, and specialists in Taoist erotic massage. The new boy on the block is able to use the Net to pick and choose from what's most appealing (and to stay away from what turns him off). He can chat with older men and get a sense of gay history and/or search out younger guys, who may be more familiar with current queer culture.

Will, twenty-three, just came out. He enjoys instant-messaging men after viewing their profiles and seeing that they are online. Some men only want to have sex (one man said he would travel five hundred miles to see Will; it sounded a little desperate, so Will took a pass on that one). But Will is amazed at the diversity in gay culture. He's met corporate types, actors, physicians, and a police officer—all through the Net. (The police officer is in the closet and needed to protect his anonymity. Will began sharing his own coming-out story with the officer, who seemed to be very confused. They continued to be in touch, and eventually became Net friends.)

One of my clients described the Net as a 24/7 bar. Just as there are "hits" in a bar, there are tons of hits online. You can "hit on" hundreds of photos, going from one to another in seconds. If you're chatting with someone you don't like, you can get rid of him with a simple mouse click.

One man told me he has no inhibitions online. In real life he works as a civil servant, in a tedious and predictable 9-to-5 job. On the Net, he meets guys and "talks dirty." He even lies, telling them he's a twenty-four-year-old lifeguard who's studying to be a personal fitness trainer. "I like the fun of fooling people. It gives me great satisfaction and for a few moments I'm beautiful and not an out-of-shape bureaucrat."

Conrad, thirty-nine, told me it's extremely challenging to meet older guys (45–55) in his city. "I don't know where the nice older guys are. They seem to be invisible." The Net opened up a whole new world of sophisticated and available older guys (though, as Conrad also said, "Some older guys I meet online are just looking for fresh meat, and that's a big turn-off").

Another advantage of the Net is its informality. It doesn't demand good grooming. You can "date" in your bathrobe and slippers.

Limitations: Cyber-Dates vs. Dates in the Flesh

Ah, the power of fantasy! Most of my clients who initially meet guys on the Net have been disappointed when they set up a date in the flesh: "He was much shorter than I expected." "I didn't think he was so old." "I thought his hair was blond, but it's more red." "He was hot in the picture, but flabby when I met him."

Kenneth messaged Darryl after seeing a great photo and profile of him on the Net. They hit it off instantly online, and spoke three hours by phone the first night. They couldn't believe how much they had in common. Kenneth was in heaven. They proceeded to speak by phone every day for two weeks, exchanging work numbers (admittedly, a little risky) and calling each other during lunch. The next step was to set up a date in the flesh. They decided on dinner on a Saturday night.

When Kenneth met Darryl, he was, to put it mildly, disappointed. "He just looked different from his picture. In my head, I had connected his picture with his voice, and when I met him, I thought I was talking to a different man. There was a nervous quality to him in person, and his laugh was way too loud. I kept checking to see if people were looking at us. Plus, he drank a bottle of wine, and I kept wondering, 'Is he an alcoholic?' "

Kenneth had created a complete fantasy in his head of who Darryl was and *who he wanted and needed him to be*. Darryl was just being Darryl. I asked Kenneth what was different between Darryl's Net picture and his real-life appearance. "His face, in person, is less angular than in the picture, slightly chubbier." I asked him what else was missing. "On the phone, I'd get aroused all the time. His deep voice possessed me. When I saw his picture, I fantasized how he'd look nude. But when I met him, I didn't feel anything. It was so disappointing. It was like the old Darryl had died and they'd brought in a replacement!" I told Kenneth to lighten up, and to remember that expectations can provoke resentment. No one looks the same in person as they do in a photograph.

Kenneth can be easily seduced into fantasy, so I recommended that, in the future, he meet guys in person within three

days of becoming interested in them online, not spend hours
and hours on the phone before the first encounter. Darryl could
have been a potential friend, if not a lover, but Kenneth let him
slip through his fingers by creating a fantasy which no one could
have measured up to.

Bradley met Al on the Net. They're both professionals in
their late forties, looking for a stable relationship and someone
to grow old with. Bradley liked Al's photo: clean-cut and conservative looking. Al had gone to prep schools, lived in Switzer-
land, and worked for Microsoft for a number of years. Now he
worked as a full-time consultant.

The two men e-mailed each other for a week and then decided to meet for coffee one Friday night. Bradley got there first,
ordered a decaf, and read *People*. Around 8:10, Al walked in, not
looking anything like a conservative preppy. Bradley was startled: Al was wearing full leather garb, with chains and a tattoo,
to boot. They shook hands, and Al went to the counter to order
an espresso. Bradley sat in total shock, feeling mortified, wondering, "What if someone sees me with this guy!" Al sat down
and began the conversation. He was very attentive, but Bradley
couldn't get beyond "the look." At one point, Al asked Bradley
whether he was into S/M. Bradley grew faint, and told Al, "No,
I don't like it. I don't care what other people do, but it's not me.
Why didn't you tell me about this, Al?" Al apologized and said
that he had two online profiles, one for the "straighter" men and
the other for the S/M crowd or wannabes. Bradley had read the
conservative one.

As Bradley sat there eyeing the exit, Al went on: "I thought
you were so hot, Bradley, and I wanted to tell you, but I

thought you'd get turned off. I wanted to tell you about the side of me that few people know about." Bradley told Al that he was not into this part of gay life. The meeting ended after fifteen minutes.

Al is not a bad guy, but he withheld information from Bradley, and that's not cool. Al's "surprise" was Bradley's nightmare. So remember: what you see on the Net may not be what you get in person a hundred percent of the time. Al thought his "hard" look might seduce Bradley face-to-face, but it totally backfired.

After Al, Bradley learned to keep his expectations low for first meetings. He realized that there are some "characters" out there, and that he ought not invest any emotional energy into someone until he'd had at least a couple of in-the-flesh dates.

Net Negatives

When we're online, we only want to show our good stuff—which is only natural. We become great editors. We know the sound bites that work. Not unlike politicians, we can spin our story into whatever is palatable to the listener. On the Net, we can control our image. In person, we can't.

There is no room for nonverbal communication online, which is crucial to any evaluation of another person. What happens when there are pauses in an in-person conversation? Pauses are essential to healthy communication. Also: What is this person wearing? How well groomed is he? Does he seem to feel comfortable in his own body? How does he smell? What do you sense and feel when you look into his eyes? On the Net you don't see waistlines or fidgeting, and you don't experience annoying interruptions of what you're saying. One man told me, "E-mail is devoid of all nuance. It's typing. You don't get the deep breaths, the sighs, the nods. I like to smell guys."

Karl is a thirty-two-year-old stock trader. Born in Kansas City, he moved to Denver after graduate school, and he's been in two short-term relationships, each lasting fewer than six months. "There's something quite appealing about chatrooms," Karl says. "I'm communicating with these fabulous guys, and we can say anything we want to one another. Sometimes I'm up till two in the morning, chatting and meeting guys for cyber-sex, but it's taking its toll."

There is nothing wrong with meeting guys online, but Karl may have succumbed to the addictive side of the Internet. I suggested that he limit his time on the computer to one hour a day, and be asleep by eleven P.M. We drew up a dating action plan, which included joining two gay social organizations and attending Unity Church, which has a weekly gay discussion group.

There are three primary reasons singles want to meet others on the Net: first is for online dating, with hopes of an eventual in-the-flesh date; second is for sex; third is to develop e-mail pen-pals. Always know what your intention is when you do the Net. If you want to date, always set a goal for yourself ("I'm going to meet three men this month"). If you're meeting guys for sex, keep in mind that it's a lot easier to have sex than it is to meet guys for dating or getting to know them. Becoming e-mail pen-pals is the best route for meeting new guys for friendship, and for expanding your gay social network.

You can utilize online matchmaking services for dating purposes, such as PlanetOut.com, Match.com, and many more. These services work if used wisely, and are an excellent means of discovering the range of gay men out there, from truckers to professors. Sometimes the number of people you can "hit" is overwhelming, so I recommend limiting your focus to five or six men at first.

You should meet a guy in the flesh as soon as possible after an online encounter, so that your fantasy doesn't rule. Do not give out your address or work number unless you feel *very* confident about the guy. You may even want to set up your date by e-mail instead of giving out your telephone number. (This is not very popular, though, since most men want to hear the sound of the other guy's voice before making even a pre-date.) Pick a coffee shop for this get-together—don't meet at home. Call or e-mail to confirm the pre-date the day before. Show up on time and dress casual/neat. Keep the first meeting short: a half hour to an hour, maximum. This is more than enough time to gather first impressions. If you feel a real connection is made, make plans to call each other the next day to set up a full date.

SELLING YOURSELF

I'll never sell my soul, but I'll rent it out.

—WILLIAM HICKEY, ACTOR AND TEACHER

The goal of placing a personal profile for the dating man is to meet a mate, not a fuck buddy. There are ads for sex, but your goal is to date. End of story. Putting together an ad/profile can be an art, because you have to be clear, precise, and concise in describing what you have to offer and what you want. For a newspaper or magazine ad, you need to be ingenious, since in most cases you're limited to 25–50 words. Internet profiles can be more expansive, so you needn't be stingy with your words; but, even there, remember brevity is the soul of wit.

Give yourself some quiet time to brainstorm and jot down ideas. The amount of care and time will be telling, because what you put into an ad/profile reveals a great deal about yourself. Be sensitive, honest, playful, flirtatious—and have fun!

Tips for Ads/Profiles

1. *It's all in the marketing:* Some men find this side of dating distasteful, but it's all about the marketing. Get yourself out there to be seen. Play to your strengths. Emphasize attractive physical attributes, degrees earned, interesting hobbies (e.g., cooking, cycling), social activities (Frontrunners, AIDS Walk), etc.

2. *Get a great photo:* Jeff Titterton, vice president, PlanetOut Partners, states that his online users get ten times as many responses with a photo as without. If you have the resources, I recommend getting a professional gay or gay-friendly photographer. Get both head and full-body shots—whatever brings out your assets. (Head shots can really show who you are.) One of the biggest complaints I get is that guys look much different in the flesh than in their photos, and that the face is not defined well enough in most posted images. Photos should definitely not be more than two years old. (A plus for digital equipment: a photographer can do wonders with it, using various backgrounds.)

3. *The shoot:* Wear something that makes you feel comfortable and good about yourself. Everything has meaning in a photo: haircut, smile, choice of clothes. Bring choices to the

shoot. You can experiment with three or four tops: sweater, button-down shirt, T-shirt, turtleneck. (Solids are better than patterns.) The most important question is: What do you want to convey? If you want to meet preppy guys, you want to be shot with a preppy look. If you want to meet a businessman, you may want to wear shirt and tie.

Seven looks
1. Preppy: khaki pants, oxford button-down shirt, penny loafers
2. Casual: dress pants, French-cut shirt, sweater, sneakers
3. Business: shirt and tie, dress shoes
4. Downtown: all black, funky shoes
5. Leather: leather pants, vest, harness, chains
6. Jeans: jeans, T-shirt
7. Hot: gym workout clothes, tank top, track pants, sleeveless T-shirt

If your photographer—friend or professional—has digital equipment, ask for a CD. If not, bring the print of yourself to Kinko's or any other copy center and ask them to scan the image at 72 dots per inch and save it as a JPEG. You can then e-mail the picture to men you meet online, or you can post it to an online dating website.

Where Do You Want to Put Your Ad/Profile?
Choices
- PlanetOut.com, Match.com, etc.
- local gay newspaper/magazine

- local gay-friendly newspaper/magazine
- your online service provider (e.g., AOL, MSN); search under "gay dating," "gay singles," etc.
- college alumni newsletter
- specific-interest organization newsletters—for example, environment/new age/yoga/attorneys/political/sports

Miscellaneous Tips

- Don't write a personal ad when you're angry or tired.
- Spend as much money for a personal as you can afford—no more.
- Anytime you're recording an introductory message for a telephone personal ad, have some notes to help you along. Avoid two extremes: sounding too extemporaneous (where you're all over the place) or too formal (like you're reading from a script).

A Potpourri of Personal Profile Words

Personals and profiles for online dating services need to be written with great skill and imagination. Here are words and phrases which may help you create magic in your ad.

athletic	tempt fate
fun-loving	sexy suitor
well-behaved	All American–type
muscular	charming
edgy	discreet
dark-featured	sports-minded
gentle soul	stable
briefs man	stylish

dork

aggressive

low maintenance

bite me!

financially secure

likes to cuddle

classy

nonstop talker

hard-core

clean-shaven

boyish

eclectic interests

country bumpkin

musical

teddy bear

color-blind

multicultural

monogamous

enthusiastic

high profile

entrepreneur

adventurous

positive

idiosyncratic

sweet-not-sour

renaissance man

heart of gold

wolf in sheep's clothing

faithful

easygoing

distinguished

cultured

down-to-earth

soul mate

upbeat

cocky

optimist

consummate

Wall Street–type

sundry

multitalented

unfathomable

domestic

angular

serendipitous

textured

devour

mercurial

refined

exotic

strikingly handsome

bookish

horseback enthusiast

culinary

philanthropic

wicked

tough guy with charm

friendship first

brains/brawn/stout heart

indulge me!

shadowboxer

hermoso

curious

uncompromising values

intellectually stimulating

self-aware

leisurely

kayak addict

picky

impulsive

magnetic

nourishing

torrid

tender

fireworks

sugar daddy

good judgment

yoga body

sugar addict

cerebral

ivory seeks ebony (or vice
    versa)

vibration

ineffable

broad-shouldered

hairy

reflective

massive

impish

eccentric

strapping

two thumbs up!

butch

iconoclast

eye-catching

jaded

proud femme

uncompromising

let the magic begin!

sweat

irresistible

mysterious

bearded

meticulous

earthy

in-the-flesh

tenacious

luxuriate

tingle

king of beasts

animal gratification

succulent

lettered

cosmic

buoyancy

moonstruck

clairvoyant

effervescent

expressive

confident

family-oriented	whimsical
bucolic	exquisite
sage	gigantic
kinky sex	soothsayer
philosophical	lean and mean

Sample Ads

HOMECOMING KING

Me: 26, 6', 175, hot Oklahoma farm boy who just came out, ir-resistible, son of a preacher, with a naughty side, MFA. Confi-dent, spiritual, versatile, tanned and toned, hopeless romantic, and great kisser. Goal: to date emotionally available men. You: 24–34, athletic, unjaded, quick-witted, and like to sweat on the dance floor.

PLAYMATE

GWM [gay white male], 30, 5'8", 155, smooth, worked-out body. Professional. New boy in town. ISO [in search of] new friends for casual dating/play; smart, humorous, adventurous, into films, hiking, and museums.

HANDSOME BUTCH DAD

GBM [gay black male], 45, 5'10", 165, lean and muscular, ver-satile top. YOU: 30–40, career-oriented, Abercrombie-type, with erotic curiosity. For dating and possible LTR [long-term re-lationship].

SHY GUYS ARE TOPS

Tall, dark, and handsome, great smile, sense of humor, passion for progressive causes, love for Jewish tradition, and a strong desire to be a dad. I'm 34, Capricorn, performing artist/teacher, attend synagogue, and am proudly gay. Enjoy jazz, films, a capella music, and country inns, especially in winter. ISO 25–40, attractive, loyal, affectionate, financially stable man, open to Jewish culture and committed to raising a child.

BIGGER THE BETTER

GWM, 31, 160 lbs., 5'10", good-looking, energetic, wild, cocky, a man who speaks his mind + goes after what he wants. Into films, biographies, working out, and carpentry. ISO gay man 32–40, race not important. Very good shape, tall, emotionally available, with sturdy broad shoulders. Knows how to cuddle and hold a man. Well-endowed a +. Must be HIV− like me and nonsmoker. For friendship and LTR.

SWEEP ME OFF MY FEET

Italian-Greek, down-to-earth, warm, sensitive, attractive, hard body, 36, 5'7", 145, financial analyst, Columbia grad. Loves dancing, skiing, Paris, museums, theater, and Tate's chocolate chip cookies. ISO 40+ in-shape professional, funny, caring, self-aware, for sensual times and heartfelt, committed relationship.

SEXY IN LEATHER

GWM, 42, 5'11", 190 lbs., hairy big bear, guy magnet. Enjoys hiking, rock music, and Stephen King. Down to earth and occasionally enjoy a good cigar. ISO cerebral, nerdy intellectual, 44–55, who yields to The Boss and can make me sweat. Also, must have sense of humor, be curious, and like to take risks. For fun, romance, and ?

Interview with Joe Windish,
a producer of Edwina.com, an online dating service

Have guys gotten married through your service?

Yes. An acquaintance of mine met his boyfriend through Edwina, and they're living happily ever after. I encourage people to use many services and generate activities that will increase their chance of meeting new guys. In our focus groups, we found that single men are looking for romance and are pretty serious about connecting for love. They already know it's very easy to get sex in the porn and sex-only sites.

Can you comment about other dating services?

Whatever works for a single guy is all right with me. I do think that some men want matching services to do all the work for them—to go out and get them a boyfriend—and they pay a lot of money for this service. I wonder what this says about a man's capability when he needs someone to take care of him like this.

Do guys lie in their profiles?

Many guys tell me, "Everyone lies." It's a standard joke among gays and straights. There's a normalization of lying in online dating, and by saying "Everyone does it," men can rationalize their behavior. Men should tell the truth. There are men who will even fabricate another personality online. What good is that, when you eventually have to meet the man face-to-face? Exaggeration and lying show a man's insecurity.

Tell me what's happening with gay men and sex online.
You can now have action sex with someone online. You hook up your digital camera to the computer and watch each other in a window. Everyone complains about online sex, but most guys have experimented with it. Some guys will swear they're going to stop, and they do for a while—and then they're back again.

What does the future for gay men and the Internet look like?
I believe that gay people, because they are so tech-savvy, are and will continue to be in the forefront of anything on the Internet online world. I read the book *The Age of Intelligent Machines* by Ray Kurzweil, from MIT, and he maintains that robots will be the next evolutionary step. I think that we may well have artificial friends in twenty years. Or I'll be able to have sex with an actual or virtual partner [online]. Or I'll be able to press a TINGLE button online and the other person will receive that tingle.

Is there age discrimination against older men online?
Older men (fifty-plus) always complain about not getting enough responses from younger men, and I tell them that most younger men are looking for guys in their [own] age range. They don't get the illogic of their complaint, because they're looking for guys fifteen years younger, [but] it's rare that the fifty-plus is looking for an older person.

TOP 100 PLACES

"Where do I meet guys?" is one of the top three questions I get asked by gay singles. Not too long ago, I would have suggested a number of bars. Though bars are still a popular place for queer folk to meet, most gay men meet their future partners outside the bar and club scene. This has been an enormously liberating development in the singles culture. No longer do men have to stand and stare in smoke-filled rooms, waiting for Prince Charming to come marching through the door.

Phil, thirty-five, owns his own landscaping business and likes to shop at a huge health-food supermarket on the outskirts of town that has always attracted a hip, New Agey group of customers, including some incredibly hot men who apparently live on tofu, green tea, and sprouts. As he pushed his shopping cart around the store one day, Phil passed a handsome man in the salad-dressing aisle who took Phil's breath away. All he could say to himself was "I want to kiss him!"

Over the course of the next two months, Phil saw "Mr. Hottie" a number of times and had the impulse to say hello, but didn't know how he would do it. He did smile at him—and the gentleman smiled back—as they made their way through the bread section. Phil promised himself that the *next* time he saw this man, he would introduce himself no matter what.

And so it came to pass. The week before the July Fourth weekend, Phil saw his man by the coffee station. For a moment, he hesitated, then said to himself, "Oh fuck it!" and proceeded to say to the man, "Excuse me. Can you recommend an interesting, not-too-strong coffee?"

The man immediately replied, with a smile, "Sure. The Mexican organic coffee has a great taste and isn't too strong. I buy it a lot, along with the house blend."

"Thanks," Phil said. "I appreciate that. I think I'll get the Mexican." Then he paused before continuing, "This is a great store. I think I've seen you here before."

TOP 100+ PLACES

An Eligible Bachelor's Golden List of Where to Meet Adorable Men

Alumni clubs

America Online personals

Antique shops/stores

Art cinemas/film festivals

Art gallery openings

Athletic/sporting groups

Auctions

Bank lines

Bars (a wide choice for all
tastes)

Beach

Bloomingdale's (or similar
upscale stores)

Book discussion groups

Bookstores

Brunch/lunch/supper clubs

Buddhist groups

Business groups

Cabaret

Campus/student groups

Catering

Charity events (gay-based, to
improve odds)

Chatrooms

Churches/Synagogues

Classical music groups

Clubs (see local gay-center
newsletter)

Coffee shops

Commitment
ceremonies/weddings

Concerts/Men's choruses

Conventions

Cooking classes

Craft fairs

Cruise ships

Dance clubs

Dating services

Discussion groups and seminars

Dog runs/walking your dog

Environmental groups

Espresso bars

Event parties (Halloween, Gay
Pride, Christmas)

Flea markets

Frontrunners

Fund-raisers

Gallery openings

Gay Games

Gay press

Gay Pride March

Gay resorts

Gay rights marches

Gay single-dads groups

Green markets

Gyms

Health-food stores

HIV support groups

Jury duty

Laundromat

Lectures

Lesbian/Gay community center

Marathons

Martial arts

Museums

Neighborhood walks

Networking/professional organizations

New Age seminars/workshops

Opera clubs

Parks

Performing arts classes (acting, dance, storytelling)

Personals

Poetry readings

Political campaigns (city, state, national)

Political organizations

Queer Stories (storytelling)

Religious groups

Restaurants (you know which ones!)

Retreats

Reunions

Shopping

Singles nights

Skiing

Special events

Spirituality groups

Stores (card shops, the mall, boutiques)

Street fairs

Subway/bus/train

Summer-share meetings

Supermarket (6–11 P.M., especially)

Tanning salons

Tea dances

Tennis clubs

Travel clubs/organizations

Theater clubs

Theater lobby

Trade shows (Gay Expos and many more)

12-Step meetings

University settings

Veterinary offices

Volunteer work

Walking/hiking

Waterfront park or esplanade

Wine tastings

Yoga classes

"I've been a regular since it opened up two years ago," the man said.

"My name is Phil," said Phil, extending his hand.

"Hi, I'm Toby."

"Nice to meet you, Toby."

Then Toby said, "Are you new in town?"

And Phil answered, "Yeah. I moved here about six months ago. I have my own landscaping business."

"Great! I own a clothing boutique downtown. I know a lot of people around here—it's a pretty friendly place."

"Yeah, I've been working on advertising and trying to get my house organized, so I haven't had a lot of time to socialize."

"Totally understand. Hey, are you doing anything right now? Because I'd like to invite you out for coffee and welcome you to our town."

Phil could hardly contain himself, but somehow managed to get out, "Sure. I'd love to."

Below, there are more than 100 places to meet guys (besides health-food supermarkets). Look over the list. Find what works for you. Be creative. Meeting men is always about taking a risk and being spontaneous, like Phil. If you're on a bank line and see a man who looks interesting, and you're not sure he's gay, you can still use an icebreaker like "Long line today," or "Short line today," or "I never like waiting on lines." See how he responds. If it's positive, you can continue with a casual conversation and see if he's really engaging you. If you feel that little spark between you, introduce yourself by first name: "Hi, I'm Norman" (the TWI!). If the conversation continues to flow, you can either say "Hope to see you again!" or hand him your number and say, "Give a call," or "I'd like to continue this." *Keep it simple.*

If you're going to a convention where you're not sure of people's sexual orientation, you may wear a small rainbow lapel pin. Other gay men will spot that immediately. Or, if the convention is casual, you can wear a San Francisco, Chelsea, West Hollywood, South Beach, or Pride sweat/T-shirt. This may cause some men to take a second look. You may want to put up a sign that says, "Lavender Caucus Meeting—The Bar—7 P.M." All of this depends on circumstances, and the degree to which you're out as a gay man.

Yoga classes are also a wonderful way to meet guys. From my experience, yoga classes are usually 70 percent women, 20 percent gay guys, and 10 percent straight men. Attend the same yoga studio/class until you get to know who's who. Strike up a conversation with a man who seems interesting: "I like this yoga class a lot, with its emphasis on deep breathing. Have you been coming here long?"

With the right attitude, and the willingness to take risks, you can let the world out there become one big dating stage for yourself and others to strut across, showing off your assets.

CHAPTER 4

DATING PROTOCOLS—GUIDELINES
FOR THE FIRST THREE DATES

For flavor, instant sex will never supersede the stuff you have to
peel and cook.

—QUENTIN CRISP

Romance is about discovering different ways of expressing, giving, and receiving love. It is a glimpse into the divine. Romance happens when two men hold hands for the first time, or when they gaze into each other's eyes and see and feel something that is beyond words. Romance may be taking in a man's scent when you first meet or watching him walk down the street after you say good-bye.

Romance means being present to each other without self-consciousness. It is letting your hair down and allowing each other to "be." For men who never want to lose control or let themselves go, romance will break down the walls of resistance. It will soften the most hardened of hearts.

Romance is not about drooling over another guy or living in some fantasy world. It is all about acknowledging another person's specialness without forgetting your own. It is two adults being "divine" with each other, in human form.

FIRST-DATE PHOBIA

Many men hate the first couple of dates with a new man. "Couldn't we just skip it and go to Boardwalk?" asked Brad. Brad hadn't been on a date in three years. He came to see me because he was date-phobic. He does a lot of excellent legwork—puts personals in newspapers and attends singles events, including gay-center dances. He showed me a list of fifteen names and numbers of potential dates, but he could not gather the confidence to call these men. Brad slips into sex "dates"—he'll meet men for one or two sexual encounters, and then end things.

I asked Brad if he would find it helpful to make a date by phone from my office, for support. He was game. The next session he brought in five names.

On the first three calls, he reached answering machines. With minor variations, this is the message Brad left: "Hi, this is Brad. I've been wanting to call you since we met at the Halloween dance last month, but I've been pretty busy. I had a real good time at the dance, and it was great meeting you. When you get a chance give me a call at telephone number _____." The messages Brad left were perfect: short and sweet.

On the fourth try, Brad reached Gary at home, and the conversation went more or less like this:

"Hi, Gary, this is Brad. You answered my newspaper ad two

weeks ago and I'm just getting back to you. I'm the five-foot-eight-inch marathon runner with a mustache and dreams of going to Prague for a weekend."

"Of course, I remember. It's good to hear from you. I was wondering what happened. You never know whether guys will respond or not."

"I liked what you said when you described yourself, that you're going to graduate school to study social work. . . . And I think we have some things in common. Are you interested in getting together for coffee?"

"Sure, what's a good time?"

"What about this Saturday? Let's see, does two P.M. sound okay?"

"That works great."

"Is Starbucks okay?"

"That's fine. I'll see you at Starbucks on Saturday at two P.M."

"Okay, see you then."

Brad was ecstatic. He ran around my office shouting, "I did it!"

It's much easier to get a date when you have emotional support. As Yogi Berra might have said, "You can't go on a date until you get a date."

But now what?

The first date is like the TV show *Biography*—except this is autobiography. You each have the opportunity to tell your story. Listen to what the other man is saying and you'll pick up a wealth of information. Remember: the one thing people like to talk about the most is themselves. You may be tempted to interrupt, or to top his story with yours. Don't. Put your tongue to the roof of your mouth and count to ten before you say a word. Let your date wax eloquent.

Some guys tell me there are men who won't shut up. Their stories seem to last forever. These men may, indeed, be blow-hards, or they could simply be nervous and trying to cover that up by talking too much. Make a decision: Is this guy nervous, but really interesting? If you'd like to see him again, could you forget about his verbosity and make a second date?

Bring a positive attitude with you. You should never bring your problems to a first date. If you had a bad day at work, let it go. If you found out you're going to be audited by the IRS, put it on the back burner for a few hours. The point of a date is to be totally present.

If, for some reason, you are not able to meet your date, call and reschedule. Say, "I'm very sorry, but something came up and I need to reschedule our date. Tell me a good time for you to meet this week." Most guys will be accommodating.

Keep your energy up on a date. You're not looking for perky/phony excitement, but the ability to carry on an animated and interesting conversation. If you're tired before the date, you may want to exercise, do some deep, diaphragmatic breathing, or take a short nap.

If you tend to create a lot of drama around scheduled events, make sure you don't rush to the date in a total frenzy, and end up in a state of chaos. Be sure to give yourself enough time to make it to the date promptly, but calmly.

If this is a blind date from a personal ad, and he's nothing like what he said he was, try not to look startled or shocked when you see him. Always remember there is a human being in front of you, and that your commitment is to have coffee for a half hour—nothing more. Perhaps you could learn something; even if he's not your type, he may be a future business contact, or he may be a potential friend.

On your first date—in fact, on your first *three* dates—do not make more than one reference to your mother, your boss, or your crazy sister—it's like bringing a third person on the date. A first date is not completely intimate—you should maintain some boundaries of privacy. Remember: you can be open with another man without giving away the store!

If your date asks you about previous relationships, just give him the facts, not all the details. "I was in one six-year relationship, which ended two years ago" is good enough. There is no reason to explain how it ended. If your date asks what happened, for now you can simply say, "It was time to move on."

If you do talk about your ex-lovers, emphasize the good times, the fun, the caring. Minimize any "drama-queen" breakup stories. At this point, your date just wants to know you're fun to be with!

One client, Sal, had been in a nine-year relationship with an alcoholic, and it took therapy and many Al-Anon meetings for him to see how his own codependency issues were partly responsible for this drama-driven union. A year after Sal left his lover, he began dating and always had the impulse to tell all the gory details of the breakup on his first date. Finally, he resisted. And after dating Morgan for a month, Sal told him about attending Al-Anon meetings three times a week. This led to a discussion of Sal's former lover which was totally appropriate, since their relationship had had a chance to become more intimate.

When you talk about yourself on the first date, be your own

public-relations department. Emphasize the good points, because this new guy is going out with you to be impressed and amused, not dragged into your lurid history of drugs and debauchery. If you went through the traditional "slut stage," skip it for now; or, if you must talk about it, or if he inquires, just say, "It was fun. I learned a lot, and that's over." End of confession.

Tell your date about your interests. What you like to do for fun. What you do on weekends. What clubs you belong to. Your religious affiliations. Where you take vacations. And ask him about his interests! Find some mutual ground! You may both be members of the local symphony orchestra. Or are you both opera or film buffs? Ask him to name his top five favorite films of all time. Ask him open-ended questions, such as "What brought you to Boston?" "What do you like best about Chicago?" "What got you interested in writing?" "Tell me about your meditation practice!" (Don't forget to sound interested!)

If your date happens to bring up a problem in *his* life, assure him about it, rather than trying to fix it—or *him*. "I'm sure you can handle it—you seem pretty competent," you can say. Then stop. You may have doubts, but he'll appreciate your support. Men who have the impulse to "fix" tend to be men who don't get their own needs met—and it shows.

I caution men about having a wandering eye during a date. If you're at a coffee shop and can see other attractive men from the corner of your eye, keep the focus on your date, no matter how attractive the guys at the next table are. It is rude to comment on the good looks of other men in these circumstances. You're on a date! For this brief time—if not forever after!—this man needs to be numero uno.

HOW NOT TO BLOW A CONVERSATION ON THE FIRST DATE

I meet guys who say to me, after meeting a guy for a first date, "God, why did I say that? It was the stupidest thing to say!" Or, "I'm so damned insensitive!"

Okay, you're not perfect. We all screw up sometimes. But there are ways to keep an open mind in conversation with fellow daters. I don't mean being a phony and not saying what you really feel. I mean giving the other guy a break.

You're getting to know someone. You don't need to act on first impulse *all* the time.

POST-DATE PROTOCOL

If the first date went well it's okay to call your new guy and talk over the phone, or leave a message on his answering machine telling him what a swell time you had, and that you'll call him again later in the week. If you do happen to reach him, and the feelings are mutual, be sure that you still keep your boundaries and refrain from engaging in a long, too-intimate conversation. The "urge to merge" is so strong with some men that, at this stage, they lose their sense of taking things one step at a time. So keep this conversation polite, friendly, and warm—and your expectations balanced.

Some men use e-mail to communicate after the first date, and this is completely acceptable. I know a couple living north of Seattle who communicated through e-mail a great deal for the first month of their relationship, and they've been together for six years. Nonetheless, I'm from the old school of dating decorum, and recommend speaking on the phone. Let him hear your

STATEMENTS MEN HAVE MADE ON FIRST DATES

YOUR DATE SAYS: I'm in AA recovery.
YOU SAY: My father was a drunk. (Ouch!)
THE BETTER WAY: How long have you been sober?

YOUR DATE SAYS: I love *Queer as Folk.*
YOU SAY: I can't stand watching those superficial queens. (Ouch!)
THE BETTER WAY: Tell me which character you like best.

YOUR DATE SAYS: I go to church at St. Francis.
YOU SAY: You're *still* a practicing Catholic? (Ouch!)
THE BETTER WAY: Have you ever heard of Dignity?

YOUR DATE SAYS: I think Hillary Clinton is fabulous!
YOU SAY: She's a bitch! (Ouch!)
THE BETTER WAY: Tell me what you like about her.

YOUR DATE SAYS: I'm a Republican.
YOU SAY: How can you be gay and vote Republican? (Ouch!)
THE BETTER WAY: I'm a Democrat. We should have some interesting talks!

YOUR DATE SAYS: I'm an actor.
YOU SAY: I'll bet you're a waiter, too. (Ouch!)
THE BETTER WAY: How did you get involved in acting?

YOUR DATE SAYS: I started therapy about five years ago.
YOU SAY: Five years? And you're still in therapy? (Ouch!)
THE BETTER WAY: I guess you have a good therapist.

YOUR DATE SAYS: I think [fill in the blank] is an underrated actor.
YOU SAY: Oh, that closet case! (Ouch!)
THE BETTER WAY: What did you like him in?

YOUR DATE SAYS: I went through a bisexual stage.
YOU SAY: Oh, give me a break! (Ouch!)
THE BETTER WAY: That's interesting. Tell me more.

YOUR DATE SAYS: I'd like to adopt a child.
YOU SAY: I can barely take care of myself—never mind a kid. (Ouch!)
THE BETTER WAY: How do you go about adopting a child?

YOUR DATE SAYS: My parents have been very generous to me.
YOU SAY: Are you one of those trust-fund babies? (Ouch!)
THE BETTER WAY: You're lucky to have helpful parents.

voice: the intonation, the resonance, and the smile that will come through. To avoid playing phone tag, give your date a *specific* time you'll be home or ask him for a *specific* time he'll be home. Don't play games. And, whatever you do, don't play hard to get.

Also, please: no roses after the first date. "But I saw it in the movies!" you say. This is *not* the movies. This is the real world, and the gift of a dozen long-stemmed roses raises too many expectations. After a series of dates, fine—but not now.

Some men love to talk to their friends about their dates, and this is healthy—to a point. Watch that you don't begin to Oprah-ize your dating, turning the whole experience into a cause for a gabfest. Be firm with your friends on what they need to know. Set boundaries. You don't tell them his dick size. (At this point, you shouldn't even *know* his dick size—unless it was mentioned in conversation!) You don't reveal something private your date told you. Some of your old friends may be jealous of your new friend, or worry about not seeing you as often as before. They could, consciously or unconsciously, try to undermine your dating progress by being invasive and nosy.

WHEN TO HAVE SEX

The first key to being a successful gay dater is: no sex for the first three dates. Cry. Scream. Curse me. But you'll see: it works.

Nate met Donald on the beach. They talked for a while and then went off to have sex in the dunes. Afterward, they walked along the beach and said their good-byes with a kiss. End of story.

Well, not quite yet! Two months later, on his way home from

work, Nate bumped into Donald on the street. There was no awkwardness. They were genuinely glad to see each other and exchanged pleasantries, each wanting to know if the other guy was still single. Nate asked Donald back to his apartment. "I want to continue our rendezvous in the dunes. I've been thinking about you a lot," he said. Donald told Nate he'd love to go back to his apartment, but he really wanted to get to know Nate a bit first, over dinner later in the week.

Nate resisted. "Hey," he said, "come up now. We can order in and watch a movie." They were both aroused. Donald said, "Nate, I'd love to go back home with you, but I want to get to know you better without having sex again right away." Nate laughed. "What's wrong with sex? We already did it!"

"I know," Donald responded. "That was different. It was summer sex with a hot guy. But I'd like to go out with you on a date this week and get to know you."

Nate was totally bewildered. He just didn't get it. For a split-second he wanted to say to Donald, "Fuck it. No sex—no date!" Instead, he asked Donald when a good time to meet for dinner would be.

Nate and Donald went on their first five dates without having any more sex. Nate has since admitted to Donald that he doesn't believe they would be together now if they had had sex again on the occasion of their second encounter.

Sex created you. It created me. It is an enormously powerful force. Kingdoms have toppled over sex. Bill Clinton almost lost his presidency over sex. Wanting sex is as natural as wanting to eat, but intimacy cannot be rushed. It takes time to know someone. Too much fast food can be harmful to the body, and too much fast sex can be an impediment to intimacy.

One guy told me that he had had powerful sex on a first date and the other guy never returned his phone call. "What did I do wrong?" I told my client that he did nothing wrong, but there may be some reasons why his date didn't respond.

First, what for my client was a powerful, intimate, profoundly loving act may have been, for the other guy, just sex, nothing more—an appetite to be indulged, so why return the call? He got what he wanted and moved on. My client was left cursing the heavens about this cold, heartless guy, but that guy was just taking care of business. Haven't you done the same in the past?

Second, when some men have an overwhelming sexual experience with another man, it brings up their own intimacy issues, and may—literally—blow them away. It frightens them. They can't believe it feels so good so fast.

There are many reasons we must take our time, and hold off on sex. Many men have told me how the "no sex on the first three dates" guideline has taken off the pressure to have sex when they didn't want to. One workshop participant said, "When I go on a date, sex seems to be the hidden agenda the whole night: Do we or don't we? Can I get into his pants? How can I get him into mine? Who lives closer? What's his HIV status? So now I tell guys up front that I don't have sex until I know someone. This gives me room just to have fun and not be thinking with my dick."

Another man said, "If I know a guy is really boyfriend material, it's easy for me to not have sex right away. In fact, if I don't really like a guy, I'll fuck him, because I know I'll never see him again—and may as well take advantage of the situation."

Dating protocol suggests that you avoid temptation and not invite your new beau to your home for coffee, or to see your high-definition TV. The home setting pulls the trigger for most guys. As they say, a stiff dick has no conscience.

What if a man really comes on to you toward the end of the date? Tell him the truth! "You're a nice guy, and I'm flattered, and yeah—I'd like to have sex with you, but I'd like to get to know you better first." See? It took only twenty-six words to say what was on your mind. Not bad! No deeper explanation needed: don't go off into what your therapist told you, or say "I read this in a book," or reveal that you're in sexual recovery, or offer anything more. You don't have to explain yourself. If he's your kind of man and the feelings are mutual, he'll respect your position. If he doesn't, let him go.

Refrain from using the word *boyfriend* even after the third date. Three dates do not a boyfriend make. It's premature and pushing it when you announce to your friends (and half the civilized world), "I'm meeting my boyfriend tonight!" Face it: you still barely even know the guy!

Be patient with the process and trust yourself. The word *boyfriend* may be appropriate after a few months or so. Keep in mind that your use of the word may even scare your friend away. Discussing use of the word *boyfriend* with the man you're seeing is a vital part of the communication process. You may say, "I'd like to ask you if you'd like us to date each other exclusively," or "We've been seeing each other for three months and I'd like to introduce you to my friends as 'my boyfriend.' What do you think?" These questions will give you some clarity as to where the relationship stands for each of you.

LET IT GO!

Meeting someone we like can bring up all sorts of emotions—feelings we've perhaps not experienced in a long time. That's why we have to honor the *process* of dating other people, and be sure to take care of ourselves. If a relationship is meant to happen, it will—without controlling behavior or even wishing it will work.

The "Serenity Prayer" works for some. Trust yourself. Trust your instincts. Trust that the universe will work out what is best for you. You've taken the action. Now, let go of the result.

Serenity Prayer

Grant me the serenity to accept the things I cannot change

The courage to change the things I can

And the wisdom to know the difference.

THE CALLBACK

One of the most frequent questions I get asked at my singles workshops is "Why doesn't he return my phone call?"

42 Reasons Why a Guy Does Not Return Your Phone Call

1. He's scared of intimacy.
2. You're not the right match for him.
3. You acted like a jerk.
4. He thinks *he* acted like a jerk.
5. He hasn't broken up with his boyfriend yet.
6. You're too good for him. He likes dangerous, unavailable men.

7. He's not attracted to you sexually.
8. He's a date hopper—moves from one date to another.
9. You didn't want to have sex on the first date.
10. You're not in his financial stratum.
11. You didn't go to an Ivy League school—he's a status queen.
12. You came on too strongly—meaning, you're a control freak.
13. You talked too much about your mother, your therapist, and your 12-Step meetings.
14. You came across as too desperate.
15. You don't listen.
16. He's afraid of your independence.
17. He's looking for a trophy boyfriend.
18. You mentioned fist-fucking.
19. You said that all religions suck.
20. He wants a sugar daddy and you're not it.
21. He fears rejection.
22. Deep down, he really doesn't want a relationship.
23. He's too fragile.
24. He's looking for the perfect man.
25. He thinks dating is a game—no gravitas.
26. You told him you have two adopted children.
27. You argued about politics.
28. You argued about Hillary Clinton.
29. You spent five minutes on your cell phone and thought it was okay to ignore him.
30. He lives in his own narcissistic world.
31. You told him you get depressed "occasionally."
32. You told him, "Size counts."
33. He's a workaholic, and dating is not his top priority.
34. He has dating panic.

35. He has an STD.
36. He has low self-esteem.
37. You started to criticize and analyze him: "You know what you should do . . ."
38. He's too full of himself.
39. You're high-maintenance.
40. You choose people who are unavailable.
41. He's a loner and lacks interpersonal skills.
42. You thought frottage was a kind of cottage cheese.

DATING AND GIVING COMPLIMENTS

A client, Brett, told me that he dated three different guys. Not one of them complimented him, though he knew they liked him.

Everyone likes to receive sincere compliments, but some guys need them more than others. It's not that they're being overly needy or manipulative; they simply need more affirmation in knowing their man appreciates them.

Compliments must feel like they're coming from the heart at any given moment. If it sounds like you're fawning, being sexually inappropriate, or looking for approval yourself, you need to back off and use better judgment.

SAMPLE COMPLIMENTS THAT MEN LIKE TO HEAR

- You look great tonight.
- I think you did a fantastic job on that project.
- You make great choices in restaurants.
- I like your smile.
- Your butt is awesome.
- I like your reviews of films—they're so in-depth.
- You make fabulous coffee.
- I like the way you take charge.
- Congratulations on your promotion.
- Your choice of wines is exquisite.
- I didn't know you could write so well.
- You do an incredible amount of volunteer work. I admire that.
- Thanks for picking out that shirt for me.
- I really appreciated your concern when my father was sick.
- You are one of the smartest guys I've ever met.
- I admire your commitment to politics.
- You write great poetry.
- I didn't realize you could sing so well.
- I love when you tell those stories about your family.
- You look great in that shirt.
- I admire the risks you take in life.
- I'm so proud of you.

TELLING GUYS YOU'RE NOT INTERESTED

So, you've met a guy through the online personals, you had coffee, and it wasn't a love connection. What do you do? What if you go on a couple of dates and it's not a match? Below, ten men explain their way of telling guys they're not interested, and my commentary.

I met a guy who I'm not sure is the perfect romantic match for me, but he's incredibly bright, funny, attractive, and is someone I'd like to become better friends with. So I told him I wasn't interested in him romantically, but I'd like to become better friends with him.

—WILLIAM

William is what I call a highly evolved dater. He tells a man he's not interested in him romantically, but in the same breath gives him high compliments and *invites* the man into his life as a potential friend. A+, William!

If I meet a guy for coffee and it's simply not working, I'll say something like, "I had fun meeting you, but I don't feel any attraction. I really wish you the best."

—FRED

Fred is clear and to the point. He can have "fun" with the guy and still not be attracted to him. Nice distinction, Fred!

It's always by phone, not e-mail. I tell the guy the truth without beating around the bush. I say, "You're a nice guy, but I'm just not interested in dating you."

—DAN

Dan tells it straight, and this works for some men. It may be too blunt for some guys, but Dan does not want to give any false glimmer of hope.

I'm one of those mousy, nice guys who can't reject others. So I write the words out on paper, call the gentleman in question, and it goes something like this: "I've had a good time over the last couple of weeks, but this is not working for me." Then I shut up and let him speak. Then, after he talks, I might say, "I'm sorry it didn't work out. Good-bye."

—JAKE

Jake uses a more sympathetic tone than Dan, but does not back off. Nice, honest response.

I'm bad. I don't call him back. I just want it over.

—RICHARD

Many men use this approach; but, unfortunately, it doesn't provide any closure for the other man. "Jeez, I thought he liked me! Where the heck did he disappear to?" If you absolutely can't speak to him by phone, you can e-mail him, though this can be impersonal.

I lie to guys, tell them I'm seeing someone else. This takes the sting out. I know how it feels on the other end.

—LYLE

These white lies are understandable, but I'd encourage Lyle to tell the truth, by phone. "You're a really nice guy, but I'm not interested in dating you."

My modus operandi has changed. I used to not return phone calls, until one crazy man pursued me so insistently that I had no choice but to call him back and tell him I wasn't interested in a relationship. He started screaming, and telling me he loved me. It was my mistake, not putting an end to it more quickly.

—EUGENE

Eugene could have saved himself a lot of grief if he had been up front from the start. Yes, there are some fragile people out there who may require a firm, sensitive, and immediate response.

I go out of town on business a lot, and this works to my advantage. I'll say something along the lines of "Look, I'm going out of town for a month and I'll call you when I get back." And I don't call back. I know it's lame, but it works. Sometimes a guy will call me again, but I don't return the call, and that ends it. The passage of time plays to my advantage.

—LIAM

Liam could have said, "I'm not interested in dating right now, and I'm extremely busy with my work," instead of promising he would call back.

If I don't see any potential with a guy, I tell him outright, "This is not working, dude." I hate when wimpy guys can't be straight with me. Sometimes, if the sex was good, I'll say, "How about doing some one-night stands when it gets cold out?" A few guys think it's cool, but most think I'm being a jerk and hang up.

—BEN

Ben's first part—"This is not working"—is great. Telling someone you're available for sex—particularly a man who was falling for you—is tacky.

DATING AND PHONE MACHINES

Part of dating protocol is healthy communication. The outgoing message you leave on an answering machine may be the first contact another man has with your home. Your message needs to communicate very clearly *WELCOME,* not *GO AWAY.* Once you give a man your phone number, you don't want to scare him away with a bad answering-machine message!

Phone Machine Messages That Don't Work

- Messages that play music before the speaker comes on. This drives most people up the wall. Who cares about your self-involved choice of music? It takes up too much time, and you come across as terribly precious.
- "Hi, this is Marshall. The weather forecast for L.A. today is . . ." I don't want to hear the damn weather forecast, Marshall—either from you or anyone! I want to leave a message! That's all!
- "Hi, this is Lance. I'm not in right now. You can leave a message after a series of long beeps." And then the poor caller hears at least twenty-five beeps. Hey, Lance: Get a better machine! Yours is annoying!
- "Leave a message." That's an actual message one man recorded! I'm going to send over some charm pills to this foolish man. Not nice. Not even mysterious.

Phone Machine Messages That Work

In this time of instant communication, your message need only have two qualities: short and sweet. Don't be long-winded, cutesy, or—worse—self-important.

- "Hi, this is Peter. I'm not in right now. If you'd like, leave a message, and I'll get back to you as soon as I can. For a quicker response you can reach me by cell at [cell-phone number]."
- "Hi, you've reached Mitchell. I'm not able to take your call right now, but you can leave a message. Include your telephone number and I'll call you back as soon as I'm able. Thanks for calling."
- "Hi, you've reached Bill. Sorry I'm not here to take your call, but I do want to hear from you. Leave your name, number, and a message of up to one minute, and I'll return your call pronto. Have a nice day."

There is a Zen saying that goes, "The way you do anything is the way you do everything." Sometimes we reveal a lot about ourselves through the smallest details, and answering-machine messages are one of those details.

NO-NO'S WHILE DATING

Dating requires good manners, wise judgment, and a healthy dose of self-esteem. The no-no's of dating will help guide you to a deeper level of understanding in your interactions with other men.

Do not judge a man purely on externals.

Get to know him! This works in two ways: if a man is totally gorgeous and just the right type for you, you may want to see what's beyond the physical form ("Hello, who's *in* there?"); on the other hand, you may meet a guy who is not very handsome but is incredibly charming and sophisticated, so allow yourself to embrace him for who he is, not a fantasy of what you would like him to be. Judging a man on externals reduces him to an object, and objectification and intimacy are mutually exclusive.

Do not monopolize a conversation on a date.

If you're talking more than three minutes straight, you're monopolizing. Come up for air!

Scott and James have been together for five years. James is the more quiet one. Scott loves to talk and is quite articulate. James remembers saying to Scott, after dating two months, "Scott, I love when you talk, but please give me a break—you're talking too much!" Scott got a little hurt, but their relationship was secure enough that he got over it.

In retrospect, Scott admits he sometimes moved from grandiloquence to being a blowhard. He needed someone, gently and lovingly, to point it out.

Don't promise someone something and not carry through.

Keep your word. When someone doesn't keep his word, it's a red flag: to keep one's word is a sign of maturity and commitment. It creates trust among people. You know you can count on the other person. You don't have to worry whether they're going to do something or not. If you have a date next Friday at eight P.M., keep the date unless a real emergency comes up. If you promise your boyfriend that you'll help him move, stick to it. If you commit to joining his family for Thanksgiving, keep your word.

Never, ever cheat on your boyfriend.

The official "boyfriend" status usually comes no less than one month after meeting, and is agreed upon by both parties. (You can actually use these variations to explore boyfriend status: "I guess we're boyfriends now!" "Would you like to go steady?" "Would you like to be my boyfriend?" "Can we talk about being boyfriends?") If you don't want to be boyfriends, that is perfectly okay, and then you can "play the field." But once you say "boyfriend," no more outside nooky!

Don't have sex with more than one guy,
even if you decide not to put all your eggs in one basket.

I encourage some men to date different guys, particularly beginner daters; it opens up a whole new social world, and gives them an opportunity to explore their wants and needs. But if you have sex with more than one man at a time, you're not dating—you're fucking.

Don't let moods rule you.

Leave your moodiness at the therapist's couch. Moods can cause instability in relationships and may be very controlling. The one thing we all want in a relationship is a feeling of safety, and moodiness will destroy that safety instantaneously.

One of the best ways to deal with moodiness is to "watch and notice" it: "I'm really grumpy this morning." "I feel irritated this evening." "I want to withdraw." "Naming" it will help you take responsibility for your behavior. Don't act out with another person.

Do not become possessive and think that the guy you're dating is a piece of property.

Fear of abandonment is the chief cause of such possessiveness. It's crazy-making, and can destabilize even a very promising relationship.

When someone becomes destructively jealous and possessive, it is imperative that they get professional help and work on some very basic, core issues, such as abandonment and low self-esteem.

Don't try to rush the relationship.

Each partner is working at his own "intimacy pace." If he starts a fight, and you think this is the end of the relationship, it may be his unconscious way of testing you, to see whether you'll stick with him through thick and thin. Remember: each of you will take two steps forward and one step backward during your "getting to know you" period.

Don't bully when you argue.

Always speak from the position "I feel," keeping the focus on yourself, rather than telling your date what he should feel, or that he's wrong about what he feels. One of the nastiest impulses in any relationship is to go for the jugular, particularly when we think we're absolutely right. If your mantra is "My way or the highway," you're going to be a pretty lonesome fellow.

Never act out rage.

Rage is scary, and can end a relationship very rapidly. Any of us may have an impulse to rage, but part of being an adult is to see the rage coming and to contain it. This can be done by immediately leaving a volatile situation and taking deep breaths—a deep breath in and a powerful exhalation. Knowing the consequences of rage can also be a deterrent to acting out.

Do not bring a surprise guest to join you for supper, or any other event.

Always clear it with your date first.

Do not constantly whine and complain.

Just below the surface of whining and complaining is anger and victimhood. Whining and complaining is very debilitating to those on the receiving end. A whiner may say, "Oh, this is *terrible* weather. It's *always* raining. There's going to be mud *all* over. It's supposed to rain for three *whole* days straight!" A reformed whiner will say, "Rain happens. Shit happens."

Do not bad-mouth other people in your life, including exes.

Bad-mouthing, whether it be gossip or severe criticism, hurts others and yourself. Talking about people in a constructive way can be healthy, but dissing people right and left is destructive. Mother's advice remains the best: "If you can't say anything nice about someone, don't say anything at all."

Don't talk about how lonely you are.

One man told me his date said, "I get so lonely. I hate being by myself." This might be totally cool to say to your therapist, but it crosses the line in an ordinary social interchange. What appears to be honesty is, in reality, dumping some unnecessary angst on your date.

Don't hold grudges.

If there's something bothering you, and you think you need to tell your date, say it! He cannot read your mind!

Not saying what's on your mind is a form of passive-aggressive behavior which can poison any attempt at healthy bonding. Ralph had dated Clive for a month, and things were going smoothly until Clive did not return three phone calls in a row from Ralph. Understandably, Ralph got panicky. "Oh no! Not another one! It's his way of breaking off the relationship. I knew this would happen!" Clive finally called, after five days, and apologized, saying he had had to go out of town on an urgent business trip and hadn't had time to call Ralph.

Ralph told Clive he understood, but he was fuming inside, and carried a grudge for the next few dates. Clive asked him if there was anything wrong. Ralph said, "No, everything is fine," but Clive knew something was up. "Are you pissed about me not calling you when I went to Santa Fe?" "A little," Ralph mumbled. "A little!" Clive exclaimed. "You're super-pissed!" Ralph told Clive that he wished he had simply called and told him about going on the business trip. "I need to know these things. I like you, and we're dating, and this means a lot to me!" Clive apologized again, and said it was easy for him to get caught up in his work and forget about other people. "But I won't do it again. You have my word."

Incidents like the one between Ralph and Clive happen in thousands of relationships every day. Some action by one mate pisses the other off, and if the conflict is not nipped in the bud, the "Big Grudge" begins. When these grudges fester, they suck the life out of a relationship. Speak up, guys!

Don't try to impress your date by spending more money than you have.

You don't have to go into debt while dating. One couple told me they spent a fortune in the first three months of wooing each other—mostly eating out in expensive restaurants. Now they cook simple meals at each other's home and enjoy it just as much.

You don't have to tell a date what your salary is, but you can say, "How about a moderately priced or inexpensive restaurant this evening?" It's a completely appropriate thing to say. You may want to impress your date, but don't go overboard! There's no room for big shots in the dating world.

Do not get embroiled in hot political/religious debates; it's self-sabotaging.

Always ask yourself the cost of going to the mat over a specific issue. I'm not saying you can't be passionate about certain topics. Keep your passion. Keep your political beliefs. The question is, are you willing to agree to disagree with a man without getting all red in the face? You'd better be, if you hope to keep dating!

Do not put yourself down.

Self-deprecation is one of the most unflattering qualities a man can possess. Some examples of self-diminishing put-downs: "I'm trying to lose some weight"—when you have a 32" waist! "I'm not great at sports"—when you swim five times a week and do yoga! "I live in this terrible town"—which is not terrible at all, just embarrassing to a few elitists. "I've never made it in acting"—when you've done great regional theater, but aren't rich and famous. "I didn't go to an Ivy League school"—but you're incredibly smart and did attend an excellent college.

Toot your own horn on a date. Talk about your accomplishments.

Don't ask, "Do you love me?"

One man told me his boyfriend nags him all the time with this, and, of course, he says, "Yes, I do love you." But asking someone whether he loves you—whether you're dating or living together—is a sign of insecurity. A better suggestion: tell your boyfriend, "I like it when you say 'I love you.' It makes me feel special." And then leave it at that. A boyfriend can never, ever give you the love that you never got from your mother and father. To think so is a delusion.

DO'S WHILE DATING

Allow Yourself to Be Vulnerable

Dating is not easy, and it can harden the heart. Being vulnerable means allowing our hearts to be broken—not in a masochistic way, but in a yielding "Take me, I'm yours" attitude to meeting a man. This requires great risk and a trust in ourselves that we will seek out and find men who will respond to our heart's awakening.

Value Friendship

Without deep friendships in our life, life would be unbearable. I tell gay singles that deep, abiding relationships with friends and/or family members is the sine qua non for any future, partnered union. No one—and no couple—can go through life alone. I tell gay men who don't have close friends to set a goal of developing five new friends over the next year—people they can call upon, and who can call upon them, when things are going great *and* when things fall apart.

Learn to Forgive

The singles life, if not approached with healthy detachment, can be a source of unbridled resentment and anger: men don't call back; someone asks if you've had "some work done"; you get gonorrhea from a man who said he was disease-free. No one is perfect in the dating world, and when dating—just as when you're in a relationship—problems will arise when you least expect them. You need to forgive yourself for not doing everything right 100 percent of the time, and you need to forgive all the rogues and scoundrels out there for being exactly what they are.

Forgiveness in no way means approving of, condoning, or forgetting about disagreeable behavior in ourselves or others. As the psychiatrist Thomas Szasz wrote, "The stupid neither forgive nor forget; the naïve forgive and forget; the wise forgive but do not forget." (See *The Spirituality of Imperfection*, by Ernest Kurtz and Katherine Ketcham.)

RED FLAGS

There are some men who, after dating a man, will say, "Why didn't I see the warning signs?" These warning signs are what we call "red flags." What appears to be something innocuous toward the beginning of a relationship may prove more serious later on.

Being in the closet is a major flag. I'm talking about men who are making no progress toward coming out of the closet, because living completely in the closet is all about secrecy and being unavailable emotionally. One closeted man told me he would go to the Gay Pride parade wearing a big floppy hat and sunglasses, and then stand about a hundred feet from the parade so that no one would associate him with it. Another man tells colleagues about weekends with his "girlfriend"; she's a woman and a friend, but there's no romantic involvement. One of my workshop attendees threw a fit when I sent him an announcement for my next workshop; there was nothing remotely "gay" on the envelope, but he said, "What if someone opened that envelope and saw a flyer for a gay workshop!" (I told him I was sorry, but felt terribly sad about people who are terrified about being who they are.) I have spoken to a number of escorts who have told me that most of their business is with "straight" married men and closeted singles.

Closeted men live lives of high drama and intrigue that can resemble the plot of a James Bond movie. What you need to say to a closeted man is "Being out as a couple is important to me. I don't want to hide my love for you or anyone. I'm sorry, but I can't date you now. When you're ready to come out, give me a call."

Does the man you are dating fail to introduce you to his friends or family after months of dating? If so, you may want to know why. Is it because he's in the closet? Doesn't he have any friends? What is his relationship with his biological family? (If they're estranged, does he share the reasons with you? A person can be highly functioning and not be in contact with his family for various reasons, but it's important to know why.)

What about promptness? Does your date show up on time or is he consistently late? Not being punctual can be a source of resentment, and this resentment can grow if not addressed very early. Randy went on three dates with a man who was late for each—up to half an hour for two of them! The man apologized, but Randy knew from his past mistakes that if he didn't nip this in the bud, it would make him terribly angry. So Randy told his date, "I need you to be on time. I can understand if an emergency comes up, but there didn't seem to be any emergencies these times you were late. I'm not waiting more than five minutes for our next date."

There can be all sorts of reasons (some not always conscious) why some men are late, but that's not your problem, and you must protect yourself from this passive-aggressive behavior. (Randy's date was on time for 95 percent of future dates. Since Randy was not looking for perfection, this 95 percent on-time rate was in his zone of acceptability.)

Does a man who lives with his parents raise a red flag for you? If a man is over twenty-five and still living with his parents, you may want to think twice about dating him.

What about a man taking care of his parents? This is tricky. Some parents may genuinely need their son's presence at home; others may be preventing their son from going out on his own, using illness as a pretense to keep him dependent on them.

Either way, I have worked with a few men who have never made a psychological break with their parents. This is crucial in achieving autonomy in the world.

Active addictions may be another red flag. These addictions may include: alcoholism, drugs, compulsive eating/shopping/gambling/indebtedness. You have to decide if you're willing to put up with someone who is "in their addiction," or if you would prefer him to be in a recovery program. Dating or living with people with addictions can provide some major drama (getting arrested, overdosing, creditors calling, family blowups)—excitement, for a while, and, perhaps, appeal to the caretaker in you—but, eventually, addictions have a demoralizing and debilitating effect on any relationship.

What about men who can't hold down a job? Is it a concern for you if your man doesn't take work seriously enough to make a living? Supporting a man for a while may be okay, but there is usually a terrible price for two men to pay when one becomes financially dependent on the other.

What about men who pull disappearing acts—just vanish for a week or two, come back, and say, "I needed my space," or "I had to work out some things"? One man—Larry—told me he had a really good dating relationship with Jeb, who suddenly wouldn't return phone calls or answer e-mails. He became concerned about Jeb, and worried about the guy. According to Larry, "Then one day, after two weeks, I got an e-mail from Jeb, who told me he was working on a special project and had just lost track of time. I was pissed! There was absolutely no reason why he couldn't have dropped me an e-mail or called me. I thought this whole thing was a little kooky, so I dropped him this e-mail: 'Jeb—I got your e-mail. In the future, I'd like you to let me know if something comes up in your life—with a call or an e-mail. This is important to me. Larry.' " Jeb responded, "Larry—sorry for not contacting you. You deserve better. Can I take you to dinner this week?" Though they did have dinner, Jeb turned out to be flaky in the matter of returning phone calls and e-mails, which Larry saw as a big red flag. So he stood up for himself. He knew he would never want to be in a relationship with a guy like AWOL Jeb.

Ricardo told Juan that he couldn't stand his "queenie" friends. Juan was a little taken aback by this, and told Ricardo that his friends were important to him. Ricardo didn't have to like Juan's friends, but Juan said he wouldn't give them up for Ricardo or anyone else. Ricardo admitted later that he was jealous of all of the friends Juan had, and of his own lack of friends, and that he wanted Juan "all for myself."

This can be a major red flag in dating: *Does the man you're dating have friends of his own, so you don't become his only source of emotional contact?* If a man doesn't have friends, you may say, "Honey, my friends are an important part of my life and you can share them with me, but I want you to go out and make your own friends."

If you feel, at any time, that you're being rushed into a relationship, you probably are. Some men are desperate to connect with someone—anyone—and lack the dating protocol boundaries that allow people to take their time and let a relationship evolve at its own pace. Some men feel, "If I don't get him right now, he'll slip away." They try to control the outcome, which usually leads to a result opposite to that intended.

One man told me a guy he had dated only twice started using inappropriate terms of endearment. ("Honey, I'll call you tomorrow!") The date would call his house and say, "Hi, it's me!" and my client had no idea who it was!

"I liked the guy," my client said, "but I thought he was being too sweet too early, and it felt kind of icky—a turn-off—and I didn't know what to say to him." I offered a couple of options. The next time that man called, he could say, "I think it's a little early for calling me 'honey,' " or "When you called yesterday and said 'Hi, it's me,' I wasn't sure who it was. When you call, please say your name until I get to know you better."

Some men engage in inappropriate gift-giving too soon after meeting someone. No one can buy a mate, though some try. Trying to "buy somebody off" comes from deep insecurity—low self-esteem—and may have a positive effect in the short run; but there's always a price to be paid for this form of bribery somewhere down the road.

John, a teacher, met Sandy, a dermatologist, though an online dating service. On their fourth date, they were walking past a store window when John pointed out a sweater he thought was beautiful. They went inside the store and John fell in love with the sweater, and said he would buy it when he got his next paycheck. On their next date, much to John's surprise, Sandy presented him the sweater as a gift, with a small card that said, "For my man!" John felt awkward accepting the gift, but he didn't want to insult Sandy by refusing it.

John didn't have to accept the gift. He could have said, "Sandy, thank you so much for your generosity. I don't want to seem rude, but I can't accept this gift. After only two weeks, I still really hardly know you, and I'm uncomfortable with this. Thanks for the thought, though. I know you meant it."

The problem with inappropriate gift-giving is that the receiver feels he *must* accept it—that there's no way out. But understand that you're not a bad man if you say no to a gift given too soon. If, after three or four months, the dynamic of the relationship changes, you can, without overstepping boundaries, proffer each other gifts—and accept without suffering qualms or guilt.

Beware of a man who wants to "fix" you. Fixers use expressions like "You know what you need?" "Let me do that for you." "I really think you should do it this way." Fixers want to run the relationship. Fixers give the appearance of being benevolent and self-sacrificing, but beware! They are usually control freaks, and control freaks are frightened people who only give off the vibe of being pulled together. The fixer/fixee dynamic is the launching pad for a codependent relationship.

Jealousy is, indeed, a green-eyed monster, which can destroy even the sanest of people. Jealousy comes from the delusion that we own and can control someone. Jealousy creates paranoia, romantic obsession, and instability—which is not exactly fertile ground from which a relationship can grow and blossom. If the man you're dating is a very jealous person, you might want to re-think dating him.

It's normal to feel a little jealous *at times,* but this feeling usually passes. It's when jealousy becomes a state of mind that takes us over or "possesses" us that we're headed toward trouble.

Charles had been dating Darren for about a month. One Saturday, they stopped at the local Starbucks for coffee. As they were chatting, a very good-looking man came up to Darren and said, "Hi!" He was an old flame, from three years before, whom Darren had not seen since they broke up. "Hi, Jeff," Darren said. "How are you?" Jeff gave him a hug and kiss.

Darren felt a little awkward, but he invited Jeff to join Charles and him, and Jeff accepted. *Big mistake.* All Darren and Jeff spoke about was their car trip across the United States, and how they had smoked too much grass and picked up dangerous-looking hitchhikers. Charles smiled but felt left out. After about half an hour, Jeff got up to leave. "Nice to see you, Darren. Nice to meet you, Charles." He shook Charles's hand and gave Darren another long hug and said, "Let's do dinner sometime," to which Darren replied, "Love to."

Afterward, Charles was livid. Darren asked, "What's wrong?" "We were supposed to have coffee together," Charles replied, "and then you invite a guy to sit with us for what seemed like two hours! And you're kissing and hugging him, and planning to have dinner with him."

Darren was taken aback to realize how jealous Charles was. He would not have invited Jeff to join them if he had known Jeff would stay so long. Darren told Charles, "No need to be even a little jealous! I had some good times with Jeff, but I have no in-

tention of meeting him for dinner. I just said that to be polite.
You're my man!" Then Darren leaned over and kissed Charles.
Charles apologized for overreacting, and admitted he had a ten-
dency toward getting jealous.

In retrospect, Darren became aware that he should not have
invited Jeff to join them, since he and Charles were a new couple, just gradually getting to know each other. If Charles had
acted out in some way (the silent treatment; an outburst) it
would have been a red flag for Darren.

Other red flags to watch out for are men who: are prone to violence; are in serious debt; are verbally abusive; won't negotiate
safer sex; maliciously gossip; are sneaky and vague in their interactions.

A well-known prophet once said that we need to balance
being peaceful as a dove and being wise as a serpent. Red-flag
alertness requires serpentine wisdom.

27 SECRETS TO ROMANCING YOUR MAN

1. Be attentive to him.

2. Take him for tea.

3. Allow your sense of humor to come forth.

4. Wear sexy clothes you know he likes.

5. Allow yourself to be silly in front of him, and vice versa.

6. Slow-dance at home—this is a high-intimacy moment.

7. Write him a poem.

8. Share astrological readings.

9. Go on a Ferris wheel.

10. Drive to the beach or some other romantic spot.

11. Make his favorite breakfast.

12. Gaze into his eyes.

13. Take a weekend trip to your favorite romantic city.

14. Find out one of his guilty pleasures—and indulge it.

15. Buy him flowers.

16. Gently rub his nape.

17. Tell him something very specific that you love about his body: "You have great eyes." "You have a fine butt."

18. Have a bottle of your favorite wine, with cheese.

19. Do yoga together.

20. Give each other a full-body massage.

21. Tell him, "You know the tongue has thirty-five muscles? Let my tongue massage yours."

22. Ask each other who you were in your past lives.

23. Buy a romantic card and mail it to him.

24. Give him a wake-up call in the morning.

25. Ask him his definition of a soul mate.

26. Explore each other's belly button.

27. Share a peanut-butter-and-jelly sandwich.

CHAPTER 5

WHAT'S YOUR TYPE?

Quiz most gay men about what they're looking for in a mate, and most likely they will begin by describing the type of man they find most attractive physically. To have a type is to have a specific preference or desire regarding the image another gay man projects. It may be an unconscious force in a man's psyche that draws him to specific types (older guys, big bears, "bad boys," introspectives, extroverts, reserved men, waifs, big shots), or a man may prefer a certain type due to cultural conditioning—the social privileging of a certain look or image which adds to and enhances its desirability (e.g., musclemen, Hollywood pretty boys, Wall Street businessmen, Calvin Klein models). Either way, types exert a powerful force on the libido.

There are those who argue that when we talk about types, we're really just talking about a man's physical attributes or external appearance. For this reason, men who are attracted only to certain types are criticized for overlooking the more internal qualities in a potential mate. But it's natural to feel a preference for a particular type of man. And most men would identify themselves as *being* of a certain type.

In the following section, I'll survey different types of men, and some common misconceptions about these types. The only caveat I offer is this: don't close yourself off from dating men who are outside your type. When you date any new person, it's inevitable that you'll learn something about yourself in the process. It stands to reason, then, that if you experiment by dating a diversity of men, your experiences will be that much more enriching and rewarding.

Your accountant recommends keeping a diversified portfolio of investments. I encourage you to keep a diversified group of men in your datebook.

What men might say about types

- He's really my type—strong, hard, and no brains.
- I like that "Winona Ryder" man—fragile as a bird and a little off the wall.
- I like those Southern boys, with the drawl and that seductive smile.
- My type is the working-class guy who is very street smart and knows how to fuck.
- I go for the Henry Kissinger type—very smart, kind of ugly, but knows he's powerful.

A partnered couple of ten years, living in Houston, told me that they sometimes joke about their types. The stability of their relationship allows them to talk about their predilections in men. Mike likes a big, burly leather man. Leo likes cute, slim Asian men. On occasion, they indulge each other's types. Leo will surprise Mike by dressing up in leather and Mike will call in an Asian masseur for Leo's birthday.

Why do men gravitate toward one type? Is it that opposites attract? Is it that we're looking for that darker or lighter side in ourselves that wants expression, but is otherwise repressed? Are we looking for someone like ourselves or who we *think* we are?

Some men may unconsciously choose a type without even realizing it: a quiet, docile man who is like their father or mother; or, in reaction to a more reserved parent, a swaggering extrovert. We can never talk about people's types without introducing the word *mystery.* The exact reason why we choose certain men—and why they choose us—may never be fully explained to our satisfaction.

Muscleman Type

Ralph, a twenty-two-year-old student, watches wrestling on television, and told me he prefers big, muscular men. I asked why. "I think they're really hot. There's something wild and impulsive about wrestlers. They don't care what they say. I can't keep my eyes off their crotches and their mammoth butts. Some of the well-muscled guys I meet are cool and detached. I like how they're obsessive about their bodies. I fantasize that they jerk off looking at themselves, with me watching them." Ralph continued, "I want these musclemen to smother me—not to hurt me, but to take me over. I want to say, 'Rule me!' " He told me he's gone out with "muscle types" and has had great times. "The incredible hulks, in person, are kind of quiet guys, and not as wild as I had imagined—but I still like being around them. I feel protected. They're like the big brother I never had. When we walk down the street, I like looking up at them."

Fatherly Type

Omar, forty-two, described his type as an older man with a gray beard, a fatherly type with a handsome face. Then he immediately said, "Oh, that's too Freudian. You'll think I'm looking for my father!" I told Omar to relax. If he likes "fatherly types," I am not going to judge him. There is nothing wrong with preferring a partner who is older or more established, financially or career-wise. Many younger gay men prefer older men, at least when they begin dating, since they feel they can learn from a man with more experience.

Businessman Type

Jake, a twenty-nine-year-old telemarketer, always had "a thing" for men in suits. "They need to be impeccably dressed, with Gucci shoes. If they're stocky, that's a big plus. Men in suits have a commanding presence, as if they have it all together. I grew up in a working-class family in Chicago, where the men always wore overalls and boots to their jobs. When I would watch TV and see a father dressed in a business suit, it seemed real strange, but a turn-on. I fell in love with Michael Douglas in the movie *Wall Street* and wanted a man dressed just like him."

Aggressive Type

Lee, a forty-one-year-old research librarian, is a quiet, reserved man who enjoys men with swagger and a take-charge attitude—the burlier the better. "I work in a very controlled environment and have a precise way of doing things. You could say I'm a control freak. Though you won't hear me saying 'shush' a lot, I do like to maintain order and to have things done my way. In my dating life, I'm just the opposite. I like the 'in-charge' guy with the swagger of a Western gunslinger, and I'm happy to take the backseat."

Extrovert Type

Some men love being around extroverts. Simon, a forty-year-old physician, is quiet by nature, and has always liked talkative, outgoing men. On vacation, he met Caesar, a thirty-seven-year-old salesman for a large computer company, whom people naturally gravitated toward. He was funny, and could hold a group captive with his charm and easygoing disposition. "I grew up as an only child," Simon said, "and my father died when I was ten. My mother was very loving, but quiet, and I spent a lot of time by myself growing up. I was always uncomfortable in dating situations, particularly when I'd meet other 'quiet types.' You could say I was a shy guy in search of an extrovert, and I found him in Caesar. He makes me laugh so hard sometimes, it hurts. When we go out for brunch with friends, I don't have to worry what to say. Don't get me wrong, I'm a great listener, and I love hearing other people talk. Caesar has a nice way of drawing me into the conversation with a question or comment."

Introspective Type

In the world of sound bites, buzz, being edgy, and appearing on top of the world, the introspective type may be considered an oddball. Anyone who doesn't seem "on" all the time may appear distant and cold. The social scene is much more extrovert-friendly. If you're outgoing, sociable, and energetic, you seem to be in the mainstream.

An artist called me one day and asked me about my work. I was delighted to take his call. He was concerned about his lack of a partner. He sounded sad, but in no way depressed or desperate. He thought he had a lot to offer another man—an assessment with which I completely agreed—but he was mystified by his inability to connect with another single gay man. After listening for about ten minutes I said, "You have enormous gifts. You have the ability to influence many people with your artwork. Let me tell you what I tell all of my clients: there is nothing wrong with you. As an artist, you require a lot of solitary time in order to produce your best work. It is not easy to make excursions out onto the social circuit and the gay-singles scene after being immersed in the creative process. It sounds like the whole dating scene is too intimidating for you. I would suggest you start taking small, consistent actions—say, one action a week—that can jump-start your love life. One action could be that you tell friends you're interested in meeting other singles." He told me that—hearing what I had to say—he felt relieved, and that he would start putting word out to friends that he was available. "I assumed they knew I wanted to meet someone, but that's a wrong assumption," he said. Soon after our conversation, this creative genius began dating a young man he met at a July Fourth barbecue. The young man very much enjoyed the company of this introspective, artistic man.

Mickey, a writer, works for a weekly alternative newspaper. He's forty-two, a good-looking guy with curly hair and gentle eyes. Mickey is an introspective man who needs and likes to spend time by himself. Some may describe him as reserved and shy, though he can be engaging in the right place and with the right people. "For some reason, people are drawn to me. A lot more people want to be friends with me than I with them. I don't need more friends." But Mickey confessed, "I want a life partner. I love my solitude, but I don't want to be alone all the time. It's not natural. I feel that if I get too used to being alone, it will become the only thing I know." I suggested a two-prong approach to Mickey's dating life: that he put together a creative profile and photo of himself for a gay online dating service, and that he place a personal ad in a well-known weekly magazine in his city, which has an excellent listing of gay personals.

Introspective men enjoy their own company. Like Thoreau, they find the examined life enticing. They're very much in touch with their inner worlds and feelings.

In the best of all possible worlds, there would be a healthy combination of introvert and extrovert in all of us, but life doesn't always oblige. So let's take each man for who he is.

DATING OUR TYPES

Jay, thirty-six, always had an eye for leather men. He got involved with an S/M group in San Francisco, and met Samuel at a "Conscious S/M" workshop in which everything about bondage, spanking, and flogging was covered in detail. The two dated on and off, and had great sex, but Samuel wanted to wait before they got too serious, since his previous partner had passed away only a year before. He knew that Jay and he had a deep commitment to S/M, so "type" worked for both of them. (They're still together. Though they have a deep, soulful S/M connection, their lives are not about S/M 24/7. They have fairly conservative jobs, go to church, and fund-raise for progressive causes.)

Jesse, a thirty-four-year-old African American professional from Chicago, likes older white men. He gets some ribbing about it from his black friends, but that doesn't bother him. He visits an "older gentlemen's" bar downtown, where mostly businessmen congregate. Though it is not populated by too many people of color, Jesse has never felt like a "minority" in the bar. "I was an only child, with a doting mother and no father. She gave me so much attention! I've always been very confident, maybe even cocky. Though I've had my brushes with racism, I've never let it get me down. I guess my mother provided a security for me that lots of other folks didn't get." Why white guys? "My first crushes were at a predominantly white high school, on the hip, white, gay students. We gravitated toward theater, the glee club, and tennis." The last time I spoke with Jesse he was dating a website designer, white and forty-four.

TYPES FROM HELL

Be careful what you wish for! Simeon, thirty-eight, a public-school teacher, was attracted to people down on their luck. If you were cute, a bit disheveled, and involved in some dramatic personal struggle, Simeon would be there to take on your cause, take care of you, and take you to bed.

One day, returning home from school, he cruised a guy who fit the above description. Lee was an unemployed security guard, 6'1", originally from Kansas City, and, yes, down on his luck. Simeon treated him to supper, and they talked for four hours.

Simeon fell in love with Lee's "tales from the street" and his Brad
Pitt blond hair. Lee was staying at a local motel and earning a
small income, he said, from selling different types of merchan-
dise on the street.

After dating for a month, Simeon invited Lee to live with
him. It was a big mistake. Simeon had no idea that Lee was also
dealing drugs, and had spent six months in prison. One day, Lee
was arrested by an undercover cop, for selling Ecstasy at a night-
club, and ended up back in jail.

Simeon had been living with a drug dealer and didn't even
know it! He had been perilously close to getting into serious
trouble himself, and possibly losing his teaching position.

There was a part of Simeon that was attracted to bad-boy
types. His relationship with Lee became a wake-up call to
straighten up and face the facts: bad boys may be terribly in-
toxicating, but they are not emotionally available. Some are like
tornadoes, sweeping through people's lives, leaving a path of de-
struction.

DATING OUTSIDE OUR TYPES

Erik is thirty-two and white. He told me his type is men of
color—especially Latino and African American men. But he recently met a forty-year-old Irishman, divorced from a straight
marriage, with two kids. He wanted my "permission" to go out
with him! I told him that while types might influence our behavior, they should never rule it. He may have desire or a
predilection for men of color, but this should in no way preclude
him from opening up to other men or types.

Jerry, a forty-three-year-old university professor, has a predilection for alternative, grungy types—guys with long hair and free-wheeling lifestyles who smoke a lot of pot. Jerry went out with representatives of his type for a year or two, with each relationship proving disastrous. He felt like he had to be an authority figure for these guys, which he came to resent. Happily, he can laugh about it in hindsight. Like many gay men approaching gay culture, he wanted to experiment, and hang out with guys who liked to party. But after about a year, Jerry began dating a social worker, who worked in a hospital, whom he met using an online service.

Sam, a thirty-one-year-old banker, was only interested in men in suits. One night, at a fund-raising dance, Sam caught the eye of a cute, alternative-looking guy, with long hair, dancing without his shirt. They smiled at each other and gradually moved into each other's sphere, and danced nonstop for an hour. Sam's friend Liz caught what was happening and yelled into Sam's ear, "Go for it! He looks like a real honey!" Sam and David alternately danced and talked for the rest of the night, and exchanged phone numbers. David called Sam, told him what a great time he had had, and asked him out to dinner the following Friday. Sam and David dated six times before David told Sam how special he was, and how much he enjoyed being with him. Sam enjoyed being with David, but his type was a businessman—not, like David, a yoga teacher and certified massage therapist. At one point David told Sam, "I think I'm falling for you," and Sam didn't say anything. All Sam could say to himself was, "David looks and acts like a young hippie. He dresses too casually. I want a conservative businessman."

Sam had to confront a situation that was getting out of control. David and he were falling in love, but David was not his type. Sam went to Liz and asked her opinion. "You say you can't meet anyone nice, and David comes your way and you just want to blow the whole thing. You're too rigid. David works really hard. So what if he doesn't wear Prada? You *like* him. What's more important than that?"

Eventually, Sam told David he usually dates business types. David reminded Sam that he had his own business as a massage therapist, but Sam said it wasn't the same thing. Nevertheless, Sam found himself becoming very attached to David, and if it hadn't been for some honest feedback from his friend Liz, Sam would have locked himself into the very rigid position of not dating outside his type.

It could have cost him a beautiful soul mate. Love is transformational, and has the power to overrule fixed notions of type. David and Sam became a couple, and have been together for five years.

There is a beautiful mystery to types. Some of us may never find our specific type, but we might find a man who meets our deepest needs.

WORK SHEET

Here are some of the types in the gay-singles scene. What qualities do you associate with each type? Do you know men who belong to each type? Ask yourself which types you might be attracted to. How might each type satisfy your wants and needs, or not?

academic	nice Catholic boy
big muscle boy	nice Mormon boy
All American	nice Protestant boy
been in jail	S/M
big bear	leather
working class	jock
older	lawyer
younger	ethereal
executive	vegan
model	actor
hipster	singer
downtown	grunge
DJ	surfer
nerdy	homeboy
European	femme
Buddhist	butch
Muslim	preppy
nice Jewish boy	

Thoughts on types

- I encourage men to date both their type and men outside their type. Don't stereoTYPE! Surprise yourself.

- You may be confused about your type and want to experiment. What would it feel like dating a nerdy guy who goes to UCLA? Or a hipster type from Seattle? Or an executive from Kansas City?

- It's possible to pass from one type "stage" to another. A friend once swore he would date only white men—until he met a charming Peruvian man in Albuquerque.

HEAD, HEART, AND PENIS: THE DATING TRINITY

Melissa, an old friend of mine, once tried to set me up on a blind date. "Jim," she told me, "you've got to meet Andy. He's perfect for you: smart, successful, good-looking, and very spiritual." I met Andy and he indeed possessed those qualities, and he was quite the gentleman, to boot. On paper, he was the perfect match for me, but something was missing and I couldn't figure it out. We went on three dates, had a lovely time, and I know he liked me a lot, but I was feeling a little guilty. I didn't want to disappoint Melissa, and I knew a lot of guys were after Andy, but what looked like a match made in heaven was only a match in other people's hearts and minds, not mine. It didn't work out, but Andy and I became good friends.

When we meet guys, there are three elements that need to be integrated before we find true love: head, heart, and penis. They're the essential trinity—one or two won't do, would mean settling for something less than satisfying. As an example, Andy worked for me in the head and the heart, but not the penis. Using my head, Andy was "Mr. Right": was an A+ person, urbane, with a great education, who went on spiritual retreats and was highly adept at managing his finances. On the heart level, Andy was a beautiful man: very kind, generous, and eager to take care of me. But on the sexual level, I felt nothing. It was like he was my big brother. On the third date he snuggled up to me and wanted to make out, but it didn't feel right, so I gently backed off. On the fourth date, I told him he was a fabulous guy who would make an excellent husband, but that I just wasn't attracted to him. I could tell Andy was disappointed—he liked me on all three levels, and that's why it clicked for him so easily.

I wish this pairing had worked, but my penis told me it wouldn't. I've spoken to many people who have had Andys in their life, and who have been Andys themselves, in other people's lives.

What might seem like failed romances can often lead to deep, abiding friendships. Andy and I became close pals, though it took some time for Andy to get over his disappointment. True friendship is a treasure and through dating—if we're open to it—though we may not find our perfect match right away, we may find friendships for life.

Head

Our head asks: Is this man right for me? Does he have the goods? Will he be there for me through thick and thin? Is he reliable, trustworthy, and fair? Would I enjoy bringing him home to my family and introducing him to friends? Does he enjoy his job/career? How's his health? What kind of vacations does he enjoy? Most of all, does he have integrity? The head takes in as much information as possible, assesses, and evaluates. Our head will ask the right questions. "Do you know you might be spending the rest of your life with this man?" Our head wisely knows that we may not find absolutely *everything* perfect about a man in a short period of time, but that as clear a snapshot as possible is important for determining whether a particular man is worth pursuing seriously.

Heart

Our heart intuits and feels whether a guy has all the right stuff. It will use expressions like: "He really touches me." "I feel better being around him." "I like his energy." "He makes me laugh." "I miss him a lot." "He's a very special person." Our heart will ask: Is he a giving person? Does he enjoy holding hands? Does he like to give and receive flowers? Is he gentle, and does he use terms of endearment? Do I feel his soul-mate potential? Our hearts may seek out an astrologer to find out if our Scorpio will match his Libra. Our hearts want to dream of a better future and live with everlasting hope.

Penis

Our penis knows what sexual connection is. We either get aroused or we don't. Our penis will know if a guy has good energy. Is he a good kisser? Is he a top, a bottom, or versatile? What about him do I find sexy: his eyes, nose, pecs, thighs, dick, butt, smooth or washboard stomach? How does he smell? Do I like the smell of his sweat?

Ideally, head, heart, and penis will agree, helping us to feel confident in a relationship. But sometimes an imbalance occurs.

When our head wants to figure everything out, overanalyzes, and insists on making things work, a healthy relationship cannot grow. Some men become exasperated while dating the "perfect guy" because they do not feel any passion toward the man. But dating is not linear; it's spiral. It unfolds rather than following a predictable course. You cannot control love. You cannot *think* yourself into a relationship.

Alternatively, the results are equally disastrous when a man falls head over heels, with no safety net—becomes an incurable romantic, prone to see only the good, none of the negative. This man may not have a life outside of romantic attachments, and may lack an adult perspective on the real world—namely, that life is not just romance and roses. Heart imbalance can make men appear desperate and out of touch, and inspires them to romantically obsess about someone who is not available.

Finally, a man may think only with his dick, limiting his evaluation of another to degree of arousal. Dick imbalance leaves one stuck in getting off and seeing others as objects.

Both the beauty and the exasperation of the dating journey is that we cannot control whom we fall in love with and who will fall in love with us. Why we connect with some men and not with others is an eternal mystery. But a truly successful dating relationship satisfies both partners in all three aspects of the dating trinity.

FIRST IMPRESSIONS

But isn't there such a thing as love at first sight, and don't all singles respond to the call of love at different speeds?

First impressions are important for all daters, but the degree of import we place on first impressions differs for each man. I have found some gay men, whom I call Hunters, know right from the start whether a guy is right for them. Other men, the Wait-and-See Guys, use a first impression as one of many criteria by which to judge a potential mate; a Wait-and-See Guy needs time to evaluate, to weigh the pros and cons of any man he meets.

Hunters are very visual. For them, first impressions mean everything. They see what they want and go after it. This is not about objectification of the hunted, but a raw instinctual reaction triggered in the Hunter's brain making him go for his catch. Hunters are guys with natural confidence who don't waste time moving in on someone. The Hunter will watch how a guy talks, moves his hands, combs his hair, moves his head, walks; the picture, above all else, is prime—a person's background takes a backseat. Hunters will use expressions like: "As soon as I saw him across the room, I knew he was it!" "He blew me away at first glance." "There was an irresistible force, beyond my control."

Wait-and-See Guys, on the other hand, need to weigh a visual impression with other information presented. Like all men, Wait-and-Sees have a strong visual reaction to others; but, often, they have had the experience of meeting and being fooled by some "Talented Mr. Ripley" along the way. (A "Mr. Ripley," like the character in Patricia Highsmith's novel and its recent film adaptation, manages to make a good impression, but on closer scrutiny he disappoints and/or turns out to be a lot of trouble.) Wait-and-See Guys take a diplomatic, tactful approach in evaluating other men, and use reconnaissance. Like a Southern belle sipping lemonade on the front porch on a hot summer day, the Wait-and-See Guy is not ready to do anything too quickly. He will use expressions like: "He looks great, but I don't want to rush this." "I've been burned before. I need to take a longer look." "I can take my time."

If a man is a Hunter, believe him when he says there's no chemistry between you. If a man is a Wait-and-See, he may seem coy, but give him time to weigh things—you need to grow on him; don't give up!

A Hunter Meets a Wait-and-See Guy

Dan attended a Valentine's Day dance at the local gay center. His eyes were immediately drawn to a handsome man drinking a soda. This man took his breath away. It took Dan no longer than a couple of minutes to summon up the courage to approach his man. Dan asked Victor to dance, not knowing it would be the start of a long-term relationship.

Looking back on their first meeting, Dan says, "When I looked at Victor, I got blown away. It's hard to describe. Not only was he gorgeous, it was the way he stood, how he looked—it was like I was watching a movie. So I just went up to him. I've never been shy in circumstances like this." Victor remembers, "I thought Dan was cute and I liked his confidence, but I didn't fall head over heels that night. I knew Dan was special, but wasn't sure if he was the one. He wanted to take me home that night; I told him it was too late, and I remember him laughing and saying, 'Too late for sex? No way!' I knew he liked me a lot, and that felt good. He was a real gentleman, and that was always an important thing for me in a guy. We had sex after two weeks, but I still wasn't sure. Dan, I knew, was falling in love with me, and he was very romantic. He did all of the usual guy things: roses, nice restaurants. I liked it when he wooed me. He was not at all bashful about showing me how much he cared."

Dan and Victor represent two distinct dating types. Dan was the Hunter, and Victor was the Wait-and-See Guy. Dan knew what he wanted and went after Victor—Hunters know how to compliment; they adore their men. Victor took his time and let the process rule, not the hoped-for outcome.

Hunters must know that Wait-and-Sees are evaluators: they will want to take a good look at you before they make any important decisions. Wait-and-Sees have developed a good "bullshit detector" through the trials of the dating world; they're patient men who want to see the whole picture.

TOPS AND BOTTOMS

> I get so tired of men asking me whether I'm a top or bottom. I
> want to say "Get over it," and talk about some real things. It to-
> tally focuses the conversation on sex, and I don't want to be
> around that kind of guy.
>
> —OLIVER, A TWENTY-FOUR-YEAR-OLD COMPUTER PROGRAMMER

The top and the bottom are perhaps the two most talked-about
types in all of gay culture. Eavesdrop on any Sunday brunch
conversation taking place among a group of gay friends and
you'll see why. "So I took him home last night thinking he'd be
a total top, but then he wanted *me* to fuck *him*! Turns out he was
a bottom."

Today, many gay men feel free to experiment with sexual
positions—moving back and forth between being a top and a
bottom—though a great many still identify themselves as strictly
one or the other. (One practical advantage of identifying as either a top or a bottom in a personal ad or online profile is that
you'll eliminate those men with whom you may not be sexually
compatible.) Despite the gains gay men have made in recent
years, a lot of misconceptions remain about the roles of the top
and bottom. In *The Joy of Gay Sex,* Dr. Charles Silverstein and
Felice Picano note that before gay liberation, gay men held
themselves more rigidly to these roles. The top was believed to
be the more masculine partner, while the bottom was thought to
be more passive.

This sort of thinking persists to this day, unfortunately.
Many psychologists have noted that some men experience
shame in being a bottom. If a boy is called a "faggot" or a "sissy"

while growing up, and he internalizes the shame associated with these words, he may feel reduced to being a bottom. (If you're experiencing this sort of internalized homophobia, a licensed therapist or counselor can help you work through these issues.)

I suggest all gay men yield to the mystery of sex. Give yourself the permission to go where you never thought was possible.

Case Study #1—Craig

Cultural stereotypes about tops are so pervasive that there are some tall, big men I know who feel ashamed of wanting to be fucked. "I'm six foot two and look super-butch to every gay man out there," says Craig, a thirty-two-year-old attorney. "As soon as guys see me they see *top,*' and I'm stuck in that role. To be honest, I like the attention—and I can get guys into bed. Sometimes after I fuck a guy and we're ready to make love again, I ask him to fuck me and he looks at me in disbelief. He can't deal with the role reversal. His fantasy of who he wanted me to be has been shattered, and he's a little peeved. One guy said to me, 'I wouldn't even know how to fuck a big ol' boy like you.' I'm just a stud to them."

Real men like to get fucked. Even my straight male friends will confess to enjoying having a woman play with their butts—with her finger or a super-fine dildo. So remember, the Craigs of the gay world are out there—men who don't want to be reduced to a certain role. Men like Craig need to be held, caressed, and, yes, fucked. Oblige them!

Case Study #2—Forrest

Forrest, a slim, 5'7", 140 lb. yoga teacher, appears to be a bottom, based on cultural stereotypes, with his soft voice, lithe

TIPS FOR TOPS

- Take your time. There is no need to rush during sex. Intimacy is about enjoying the moment.
- Take the pressure off yourself to "perform," to be hard all the time. Some men naturally remain hard for a long time, others' erections come and go. There is nothing wrong with tops who can't maintain a constant erection. Get rid of the notion that you're a stud who can fuck at the snap of a finger. If you do go soft, allow yourself time to get hard again—it's not a contest; you're not being clocked. If you don't get hard during a lovemaking session, that is okay, too. Using your ingenuity, you can still have a hot time.
- Ask your man how he likes to be spoken to during lovemaking. Whispered sweet nothings in his ear as you play with his butt? Wild, dirty talk that brings out the animal in both of you?
- What do you want your partner to say to *you*? Tell him. Bottoms are not mind readers. They need to know the wishes and wants of their tops. "Tell me to fuck you hard!" Now, that's being specific!
- Ask him if he wants his asshole massaged before penetration. Always have lubricant ready. Be gentle.
- As you're entering him, you can say, "How does this feel?" "Are you okay?" "Let me know if you want it harder." "Is it too much?" "I'm with you, baby." Communicate. Don't assume anything.
- Have a condom within reach at all times.

dancer's body, and sensitive nature. Forrest also has a determined, competitive side to him that not too many people see. Forrest enjoys fucking men, though some find this to be a bit of a shock. "I fool guys and get a kick out of it. Some guys can't figure it out, and I love the confusion because it creates some interesting sexual tension. 'You're going to fuck me? No way!'

TIPS FOR BOTTOMS

- Tell your man what you like. Do you want him to be gentle? Do you like it when he takes over and surprises you with his manliness?

- If, at any time during your lovemaking, you want your partner to stop, tell him! You don't owe him anything. It's imperative that your partner respect your limits.

- If your partner is not hard all the time, this is perfectly natural. It doesn't mean you're not sexy. Don't make him too self-conscious, by trying to get him hard again immediately. He might need some time to "hang out" with you in bed before he gets back to business. Men love their penises! Play with his and tell him how much you want him.

- Ask your man what he likes to hear during lovemaking. He may want a lot of dirty talk or simply to take in the moment in silence.

- If your top is a little nervous, tell him he's doing really well. Say, "That's great, baby!"

When they see I'm for real, they get into it and we have some pretty hot sex. I don't limit myself. If I get good vibes from a guy and he's sensitive, I don't mind at all being a bottom."

Frequently Asked Questions

What happens when two tops or two bottoms date each other?
Some men consider themselves exclusive tops or bottoms, meaning they are unwilling to change sexual roles. These exclusives need to state early (though not on the first date!) what they prefer in bed. If someone is exclusive, don't try to change him. (This can become a power game. One top I worked with was dating another, and they had sex without penetration, though each one was

hoping that the other would give in. So it became a game of "Who's going to give in first?" These sexual games are not healthy.)

Two bottoms in a dating situation can be problematic, too. It's especially difficult if each man really wants to get fucked, but neither wants to oblige the other.

I agree with the therapist Michael Schroeder that exclusives are placing themselves in rigid sex roles and not allowing for spontaneity. I don't try to change exclusive tops and bottoms, or shame them into doing something they do not want to do, but I do ask them to look into the feelings that come up for them about reversing roles in bed.

Some tops are so culturally conditioned, they wouldn't dare consider getting fucked. But if they have an opportunity to talk about the feelings that come up around penetration, some—though not all—reconsider their options in bed. Some tops are scared of being the receptive partner simply from fear of the unknown. One guy told me, "I never thought about being a bottom, because I thought it would hurt"; but one day he was with a guy who was totally hot and knew his way around "the land down under," and my client gave himself completely—and was glad he did!

Exclusive bottoms may not have even thought it possible to be a top. Maybe they feel they're not "man enough," or that they don't have a big-enough dick, or perhaps they worry about maintaining an erection. I recommend communicating your feelings to your partner—telling him, if you're primarily a bottom, that you would enjoy reversing roles sometimes. Good communication is the sine qua non of good sex.

How often should my partner and I have sex?

Each couple is different and will approach their sex life differently. I know beginning couples who have sex every day. I know couples who've been together for fifteen years who have sex once a week. There are couples who get into a routine of kissing, hugging, and jerking each other off. I know of a couple together for nine years who have long, passionate sex two or three times a month. I know some couples who switched top/bottom roles after three or four years.

Find what works for you as a dating man, and what works in a committed relationship. If the need arises, talk to your therapist or support group about the issues that most concern you and/or your partner. If you feel it's appropriate, you may want to seek out a certified sex therapist or counselor to discuss any problems you and your boyfriend may be experiencing.

Is it possible to have anal sex without it being so complicated and messy?

Having pleasurable and intimate anal sex may take time for some men. One of my clients who visited an escort recounted how surprised he was that the hour went by so smoothly.

There's an old joke: "Do you know how to get to Carnegie Hall?" "Practice, practice, practice."

The same might be said of anal sex. The escort practices anal sex, and wants to please his customer. Though our dates and boyfriends are not customers, we certainly can learn the skills used by an escort in our own bedroom.

Though I do not want to endorse escorts as a primary means of getting one's sexual needs met—particularly for men in sexual recovery—I think an experienced and conscientious escort can provide a valuable sex education for some men.

INTERVIEW WITH AN ESCORT

I interviewed Angelo, a twenty-eight-year-old escort, about what he's learned about gay sexuality. Here are some of his thoughts on sex and intimacy:

Erogenous zones

"Find your man's erogenous zones while you're making love. Is it working his nipples? His tongue? Playing with his asshole? Kissing the side of his neck? Each man is different, so find his zones of pleasure. Watch your partner. What makes him groan? When do his groans get louder? Making love is about passion, so be passionate about what you're doing. It's not just 'in and out.' "

Anal sex

"If you are going to be a top you *must* take your time. You're putting something in there besides your dick. Make love to him. Kiss him. See if he's comfortable. He must be *relaxed* before you enter him. Massage his anus with your finger for forty-five minutes, off and on, so he wants you to fuck him, so he's totally relaxed. You both need to be in the mood. I cannot recommend rimming, because of the risk of contracting parasites or hepatitis, but it certainly helps a man to relax. If you know someone who is STD-free over a long period of time—and you trust him—this may be an option."

Supplies

"Always have condoms, a towel, and a lubricant nearby. I use Eros lubricant, because it doesn't get sticky."

Metamorphosis

"I massaged an exclusive top's asshole off and on for almost an hour, and he groaned, 'Fuck me.' I've known bottoms to become tops when they see a man who wants to get fucked. It's all in the head."

Bottoms up

"If you're a bottom, make sure you have a clean asshole. You can keep your anus and rectum clean with a high-fiber diet."

Viagra

"I use Viagra sometimes to ensure performance. But you have to be careful you don't get hooked on it. My doctor told me Viagra causes a potentially fatal drop in blood pressure when combined with the nitroglycerin that some guys use for heart disease, or poppers for sexual stimulation."

Foreplay

"Foreplay is crucial to good lovemaking. Get your partner in the mood. Start with gentle kissing. I watch men melt in my arms after I put my mouth to theirs. Don't set a time in your head for how long you're going to kiss. One of my clients practically orgasms when I kiss him. He writhes and clutches me. If it feels right, I will gently breathe into him, like I'm giving artificial respiration. Deep emotions are triggered by the gentle exchange of tongues. Don't just stick your tongue in. Slowly tease. I see a tongue as another penis, ready to stimulate and be stimulated. Make sure you're touching your partner while kissing, slowly moving your hands across his body. Look into his eyes and at his face. The expression on his face should tell you whether you're hitting the right spots."

CHAPTER 6

KEEPING A HEALTHY
BODY AND MIND

Many of the men I meet in my practice speak about the enormous pressure that exists in gay culture to look perfect—to achieve the perfect, chiseled body. It's no wonder. Each day we're bombarded with images—on billboards and in magazines, on the Internet and on television—of men with physiques that have been rigorously developed. But developing a body that's fit to appear on the cover of *Men's Health* is beyond the reach of most men. The writer Michelangelo Signorile has written about what he calls "body fascism" and its hold on the gay male psyche: "Body fascism can perhaps be defined as the setting of a rigid set of standards of physical beauty that pressures everyone within a particular group to conform to them. Any person who doesn't meet those very specific standards is deemed physically unattractive and sexually undesirable." The pressure to look perfect in the dating world can be enormously stressful, and take the fun out of dating. If a man is constantly evaluating himself against

the impossible, supposed norms projected by mainstream culture, his self-confidence will always suffer.

Eric, a twenty-three-year-old graduate student, told me
about his journey as a gay man, which began during his college
years. "I grew up in a suburb outside Denver and knew I wanted
to attend a university with a large student population, a place
where I could be anonymous. I buried myself in vigorous aca-
demic work and all but forgot about a social life. I made dean's
list and was shooting for Phi Beta Kappa. It wasn't until my third
year in college that my personal life took an unexpected turn. I
was forty pounds overweight, so I met with a nutritionist on
campus who put me on a balanced food regimen and enrolled
me in an exercise program. It took a year and an extraordinary
amount of discipline, but I finally achieved the body I always
dreamed of having. I found out that being in top physical shape
not only got me attention which I had never gotten before, but
that guys would actually come on to me." Eric achieved status
and recognition, which he craved in his teenage years but never
got, due to being overweight. But soon, losing the extra weight
wasn't enough. Eric wanted to have a body like the ones on the
covers of men's fitness magazines.

Eric cultivated the "body perfect" persona. He realized that
his Phi Beta Kappa key had less status in gay-single life than
being in top physical shape. I suggested to Eric that he consider
setting aside time each week for activities outside the gym, such
as community-service work, or joining an extracurricular group
to develop his leadership skills. While there's nothing wrong
with wanting to develop a better body, when a gay man sees a
beautiful body and doubts his own attractiveness, he succumbs
to "compare and despair." Remember: your success as a dater, in

the end, will depend more on the internal qualities that you develop than on your external appearance. So don't just spend time at the gym. Take up a hobby. Read a book. Go see a film with friends. You owe it to yourself, and to your future boyfriend, to be as interesting a guy as possible.

Mary Florence, a counselor from a local university, called and asked if I could come and speak to gay college men, ages nineteen to twenty-four, on the topic of body image and self-esteem. She told me that she was concerned that many young gay men were becoming obsessed with their bodies—some becoming anorexic and others trying to become Mr. Atlas by abusing steroids. Mary Florence also works with straight women, and related that she found some startling similarities between straight women's and gay men's attitudes toward body image. "Am I beautiful enough?" is the number one question on their minds—male or female.

The college attendees at the workshop were an extraordinary group of men. I started the evening's event by asking them what feelings came up for them around body image in the gay community. Kevin, a third-year science major, told the group that he felt a lot of anger. "Look, I go to bars and no one, absolutely no one, looks at me. I don't think I'm bad-looking. I do get a couple of beefy older guys who think they have the right to grab my ass, and I tell them to fuck off. But I'm angry. I keep thinking, What can I do? I know I don't have that perfect body, and I'm twenty pounds overweight, and I think maybe I need to go to the gym more often. My fear is that I'll lose the extra poundage, come back, and still get ignored."

Drew, a communications major, felt confused. "I think I look like a nerd, and I'm attracted to nerds, but I'm not sure if

I'm attracted to nerds because I think they're the only guys who would find me attractive." I asked Drew if he would agree to my asking the group if he looked like a nerd or not. He said sure. In that group of men, no one thought he looked like a nerd.

Like Drew, many men will label themselves out of fear and a sense of isolation. Drew began to internalize the notion that he was a nerd, which undermined his confidence. Remember: there are bookish librarians whom some men find very attractive. There are guys who are self-conscious about a body scar that other men might find sexy. Sometimes what we despise about our own bodies are the very things other guys find attractive. Will Smith has big ears, and many people find him very attractive, ears and all! Actor James Woods is not handsome by Hollywood standards, but is very sexy to quite a few men and women.

The lecture brought home to me the extent to which young gay men today are confronting a body-image-obsessed culture. They looked like all-American guys (albeit from different cultural backgrounds), each of whom would make the perfect boyfriend. But underneath the engaging cockiness of youth were men starting to doubt their self-worth. And the thought of mainstreaming into gay culture after college scared them immensely. I encouraged the group to cultivate friendships with other gay men and lesbians, so that there will always be the presence in their lives of people who know, at the deepest level, what it means to be gay.

Pick up any gay magazine, or Abercrombie & Fitch catalog, and you'll find 99 percent of the men shown to be beautiful beyond imagining. It is hard to compete with such beauty. It's too easy to look at yourself in the mirror and say, "God, I wish this part of me could improve! Because if I don't improve, I won't find the man of my dreams!" I do not suggest that we stop reading magazines, but that we do be aware that we're looking at models—a very select group of men whose vocation is their appearance and who have the added assistance of great lighting and make-up artists.

At my workshops, when I ask gay singles to write down their internal qualities—like loyal, well balanced, sensitive, caring—they can do it quite easily. When I ask them to write down external qualities—like beautiful eyes, handsome face, and nice physique—they are a lot more resistant. When I ask them to break into pairs to discuss their qualities with another man, they balk at detailing their physical qualities. "I hate to tell another gay man that I'm cute," one man confessed. I asked why. "Oh, it just feels funny. I get embarrassed, because he might say, 'Who are you to think you're handsome?' " I tell the paired participants in my workshops not to comment on each other's listing of physical qualities, because the purpose of the exercise is to become better able to verbalize these qualities in front of another man—and, to do that, it helps to be heard without judgment.

Like Kevin and Drew, above, gay men need to feel safe when they talk about body image. They need to feel that they are not going to be attacked or made fun of. Many men did not receive "body validation" as young people, and many gay men are starving for such validation. For years, gay men used sex as a temporary means of obtaining approval; but can you imagine how validating it would be for a gay man to hear from his father, "Son, you're a handsome boy. You're going to make some guy very happy someday"? I often say to clients, "You're a really good-looking guy," and I mean it. Maybe it's because I'm older than many of them, and/or that they know me well enough, but my clients don't feel embarrassed by the compliment or think I'm acting inappropriately or being disingenuous.

We've all been in situations in which we doubt our attractiveness. There are men who will leave for a social event, come back feeling that they're not good-looking enough to go, and stand in front of the mirror judging themselves mercilessly. I can tell a man one million times he's good-looking, but if he doesn't absorb that compliment—truly take it in—he'll still think he's unattractive. And—trust me—if you keep telling yourself you're not attractive, you'll begin to believe your own lie. Your inner teenager is scared—he needs encouragement and support. You need to release the old, worn-out mind tapes of self-criticism and access that part of you that is loving toward and confident in yourself. Guys like confident men!

Whenever a man is feeling shame about his body, I recommend that he seek out a good therapist, to whom he can verbalize his feelings about body image in a safe environment. Some of my clients find it excruciatingly difficult to speak about their bodies; but, when they do open up, an enormous weight is taken off their shoulders.

DICK SIZE

Bud is terribly embarrassed about his dick size. He feels inferior to other guys, and was terrified about taking showers in high school. He even investigated some of the ads on the Internet promising penis enlargement, but decided against it. I told Bud that most men I talk to consider dick size icing on the cake, and are more turned on by a date's other external and internal qualities. When Bud started dating—not just having sex—he met a different class of men: guys who could see beyond dick size.

We live in a society that quantifies everything to an extreme, so why not dick size? Yes, liking a big dick is perfectly normal, but obsessing about getting or having a big dick can be a major waste of time, energy, and even money, if one goes for penis enlargement "treatments," which are nothing more than scams.

We get a distorted idea of penis size from pornography, where all the dicks appear to be twelve inches, or from folklore: "This guy I met had the biggest dick I've ever seen—ten inches!" The average erect dick has a normal range of five to seven inches. If you have a smaller dick, there's no reason to put yourself down, like Bud. If you happen to have a big dick, it's no reason for feeling superior to other men, nor for indulging the thought that guys want you *just* for your dick size—that's their issue, not yours. (It's also inappropriate, not to mention tacky, to volunteer your dick size without anyone asking.)

Though some advertisers of penis-enlargement kits promise you a bigger dick, my advice is to leave well enough alone: to take pleasure in your penis, whatever its size or shape, whether it's cut or uncut.

Tips on Dick Size

- Stop worrying about it. Most gay men will tell you that dick size is only one aspect of a gay man's sexual makeup. It's the total package that counts.
- There is no need to apologize for your size before, during, or after you have sex. This is a big turn-off.
- If it feels right and you have a trained group leader, talk about your dick size in a gay support group. A lot of shame can be lifted by speaking honestly about your feelings.
- Check out David M. Friedman's book *A Mind of Its Own: A Cultural History of the Penis.* Your penis has a history, so ap-

preciate your dick—whether small, medium, or large—in its historical context!

DEALING WITH BODY-IMAGE ISSUES

There is a lot of shame associated with body image. Some younger men are worried about being wrinkled at age thirty-five. Older men feel no one is even looking at their bodies; they feel totally invisible. Very young men feel that there is something wrong with their bodies—that they are too skinny or fat, too short or tall—and that they must do something with their bodies (anything!) to get a better look, so that more people will pay attention.

One client, age thirty-nine, worried about his gradual hair loss and asked me whether he should get a hairpiece. I told him that I could not give him a yes or a no, but I could discuss the pros and cons with him. He hated the idea of being bald, because he thought it would limit him in the dating scene. I told him that some guys aren't attracted to bald men, but others find them sexy, and still others look at the whole man, to see whether there's a connection or not.

Nevertheless, he wanted to do something about it, and said, "I don't want to make it look so obvious that it becomes laughable!" I told him that he could find some excellent hair-replacement centers whose work might surprise him, and that the most important thing about a hair replacement is that it look and feel like it absolutely belongs on your head. (With high-quality hair replacement, you can live your life quite naturally, without fear of detection—and can relax when you have sex—because your new hair won't come off.)

Having looked at both sides of the issue, my client decided to get a hair replacement. It did look fabulous, and I believe it helped him gain more confidence in the singles scene. (At some point, though—I recommend sooner rather than later—you should tell your partner about your hair replacement. If a man really likes you, this will not be the determinative factor in whether he stays with you or not. Trust him. Trust yourself.)

Some guys I know impulsively shave their heads, looking for an edgy "in" look. One stylist told me that a shaved head looks great on a young man who is in excellent muscular condition as well as on men of color. Speak to your hairstylist first before making any radical changes—he or she may be able to help you pick the most flattering cut.

We've examined how body image plays out in gay culture and why gay men must confront this issue head-on if they want a place at the dating table. So: What about joining a gym, and getting or staying in shape?

Jack, a thirty-seven-year-old marketing executive who is slightly overweight, was fed up with the emphasis on the perfect body in gay culture. "Why are gay men so obsessed with looks? Can't they see me, *me*?" I asked Jack if he was comfortable with his body and he said no, but continued criticizing "those queens out there."

I said, "Jack, you're living in a city with a large gay population. If you say 'To hell with it—that's who I am,' I understand, but most men are visual and make assessments." Jack thought he could take the easy way out and not get in shape. But I think men dating men need to take an honest look at themselves and ask whether there's anything they need to do to enhance their physical appearance. Perhaps it's joining Weight Watchers, going to the gym, or walking in the park for a half hour every day. Being a well-groomed, in-shape man is all about self-respect and healthy self-image, not about body obsession.

But, then, when does gym life become too much of a good thing?

Some men become addicted to gym life because they want the perfect body, and they'll compulsively keep looking into the mirror, both at the gym and at home, for one more imperfection that needs to be corrected. One hour of working out becomes two or three hours, in hope that a Greek god will appear in the mirror.

Looking like a Greek god is wonderful, but if a man's life becomes consumed with *only* the external, he'll *never* feel satisfied. He'll end up wandering the dating world as a half person.

Cosmetic Surgery and Dating

Dermatologists will tell you there are gay men in their thirties coming in for cosmetic surgery. Once some guys see those first wrinkles, it's off to the dermatologist for a consultation. One dermatologist told me about a twenty-three-year-old actor who asked to have work done to remove his laugh lines—so he would be considered for younger roles!

One doctor told me that he has advised some men against cosmetic surgery, knowing that what they really needed was reassurance that they looked just fine as they were. "One patient was convinced that his lower lip was too small and needed augmentation, but I said it looked perfectly okay to me. He left my office feeling a lot better."

If you do decide on cosmetic surgery, know that the dermatologists I have surveyed told me that most men are satisfied with their work. With a skillful surgeon, such work is undetectable.

Some general comments about getting "work done":

- Seeking out cosmetic surgery is a very individual choice. Some men may think they need cosmetic work. Others accept who they are and may even take some pride in looking older, considering cosmetic surgery an exercise in vanity. Some men won't consider it simply because the cost is prohibitive.
- Some men, due to some deep insecurities about who they are, may need to see a therapist more than a dermatologist. A few men may have a psychiatric disorder: BDD—Body Dysmorphic Disorder. Such a person hates his body and will compulsively seek out ways to change how he looks. (A good dermatologist will refer him to a psychiatrist for treatment.)
- It helps to have a good rapport with your doctor in making decisions about cosmetic work. He/she can gently ask:

  1. How did you hear about cosmetic work?
  2. What are your expectations? (Looking thirty years younger is not realistic. Looking "relaxed and healthy" may be.)
  3. Do you know the risks? If you don't, ask your doctor what they are. Also, he/she should know your medical history.

- The doctor must know if the patient has any concerns. As with all medical procedures, there must be trust between the patient and surgeon.

• Gay men should do four things in exploring cosmetic options:

1. Talk to friends. Your good friends may be persuasive enough to convince you of your own attractiveness, without the need for cosmetic surgery. Listen to them!
2. Use the Internet as a source of information. Some doctors have great websites, but you will also want to have a number of questions prepared for the in-person consultation.
3. Talk to two physicians—get a second opinion.
4. Become a "knowledgeable consumer." Do plenty of research before deciding on a course of action.

Interview with Richard A. Marfuggi, M.D.,
author of Plastic Surgery: What You Need to Know

What types of procedures do men come to see you for?
Some will come in for treatment of male breast enlargement, in which the breasts look like a woman's, which can cause deep embarrassment. I have found that men in their late teens will want work done on their noses, or need skin care due to bad acne. Men in their twenties tend to be looking for body contouring or want to have bags removed from under their eyes. They're very much into body image. This is also the age at which I begin to get requests for liposuction, which is also popular for men in their thirties. Men in their thirties will also come to me for work around their eyes, due to aging. Gentlemen in their forties and fifties come to see me for chin, neckline, and jowls. I have a

"weekend face-lift" just for the jowls. Men who are over fifty might consider a face-lift. Guys in their sixties, seventies, and eighties come for wrinkles or skin treatments, like a chemical peel.

Are there quacks out there?

Absolutely. Though the vast majority of plastic surgeons are highly competent, there are unscrupulous people who will say they are plastic surgeons but are not. There was a case of a dentist from Venezuela doing plastic surgery. Newly arrived immigrants can be easily duped by misleading advertising. You must check out the credentials of the health-care professional, and make sure that he/she is a board-certified plastic surgeon.

Do you work on men who are HIV+?

Yes, I do, but I always check with their primary physician so I don't compromise their health. We must know all the prescribed drugs they are taking, plus herbal supplements. One man was taking twenty-three supplements! Remember: herbal supplements are drugs, and some of these drugs can affect a patient's blood thinner, which in turn affects his recovery from bleeding.

Can cosmetic work help men get dates?

Cosmetic work can change the look of a man, but not his personality. Some men will have their ears, belly, and nose worked on and still not get a date, because—basically—they're not nice people. I can change a man's look, but I cannot turn him into a different person.

Do you think having work done is a refusal
to accept getting older?

It can be. I tell men never to lie about their age, even after they have plastic surgery. If you're forty-five and look ten years younger [because of surgery], tell people you're forty-five and, in the vast majority of cases, they'll say, "My God, you look much younger! I would never have guessed it!"

Body-Image Solutions

1. Be aware of the cultural conditioning that hits you every second in modern society. How much do you want to buy into the perfect-body syndrome? Looking fabulous is important, but going overboard and becoming consumed with your looks is not healthy. Nowhere is moderation needed more for gay men than in the concern over body image. You don't have to feel lousy about yourself (one extreme) or superior to everyone else (the other extreme). You can look fabulous without losing your heart. Don't be "addicted" to extremes. Live a life of moderation.

2. If you become obsessive about your looks and compulsively work out or search for the latest magic potion, it's time to take up other activities that will nurture your spirit. Your Saturday does not have to be consumed with the gym and working out. How about reading that latest bestseller that you've been putting off, or joining a club, or taking a class in cooking, Spanish, or dance?

3. For some gay men, the gym is a social outlet, which is great—but I challenge you to broaden your outlets. How about joining a softball, basketball, or soccer league, which almost always have games on weekends?

4. Volunteering can be a means of taking the focus off of yourself. What about volunteering at an HIV-prevention program, a legal-services organization, Meals on Wheels for the elderly, or a gay-youth empowerment project?

5. Get help if you need it. Reach out to other people if your life seems a little out of control. If you're suffering from PBS (Perfect Body Syndrome), which can produce a lot of anxiety, and you're harming yourself by excessive dieting, bingeing and purging, or any other eating disorder, please seek out professional help by contacting www.nationaleatingdisorders.org or calling (800) 931-2237.

DATING AND HIV

Body image and HIV go hand in hand. HIV+ men tell me all the time that one of their biggest fears is not being desired again by another man. Hence, the impulse to stay ignorant or silent about status. Who wants to feel they're not being looked at and admired?

Conscious dating and the establishment of long-term, intimate, satisfying relationships is one of the best means of prevention of HIV. Conscious dating means getting to know someone before having sex. It's about forethought and making good judgments when it comes to situations that have the potential to harm or hurt us.

Some gay men are beginning to see that the paradigm shift in dating involves getting to know someone before having sex. This is not a puritanical notion. Rather, it is about delaying short-term pleasure for a long-term goal (a relationship). It's a given that we all want to have sex—a biological drive which created six billion people on this planet—but it should not prevent us from looking HIV in the face and examining our attitudes toward safer sex, whether we're Poz, Neg, or not sure.

Self-Examination

Some gay men are starving for affection, and will do anything to satisfy this hunger and allay their loneliness, even engage in unsafe sex practices. It's crucial that you develop a support network—whether it be friends, a church community, or 12-Step fellowship—that provides you with affection and love.

There are men who feel that their worth is defined by being in a relationship; that, without a boyfriend, a big hole exists in their lives. In this context, desperation can set in and a man can easily give his power away. Giving our power away means that clear, rational thought is discarded for the sake of pleasing someone else. We lose our sense of self and reason. This loss of self can be exhibited through masochistic and self-destructive acting out. Some men suffer from deprivational thinking, which sends signals to the brain suggesting we're never going to get what we want unless we get it now. (Because of this, I tell men never to put themselves in compromising situations, such as inviting a man home on the first couple of dates, since this can so easily lead to sex.)

There are millions of people in large urban areas, and yet many are lonely. Why does this have to be? If we have the right attitude—are open to meeting new people—many friends will appear in our life; but, if we whine and engage in deprivational thinking ("Poor me. There aren't any good men around"), our lives will be loveless.

Deprivational thinking is claustrophobic, and deprives us of a world of possibilities and abundance. It tells us, "Settle now, because there's nothing else out there." But in no circumstances should we settle for unsafe sex!

Some men have sadistic tendencies; they could care less about hurting another person through unsafe sex practices. Some are codependent; they feel compelled to fulfill what another person needs and wants, no matter what, instead of paying attention to their own needs and wants.

Expressing clearly to men that we don't want to have sex right away—and negotiating safer sex—may seem simple enough to do, but it's certainly not easy. Sometimes the words get caught in our throat and we just can't get them out. Why? Many of us just want to be liked, and the fear of rejection is too overwhelming. Or we didn't learn the art of clearly communicating while growing up. Here are some statements you can add to your dating tool kit for use when the occasion arises.

Holding Off on Sex

- "It takes me time to get to know someone before I have sex."
- "I really like you, but I don't want to have sex tonight."
- "I think you're hot and I want to fuck, but let's hold off for a little while."
- "Let's go for a walk instead of going back to your place."
- "I know it's old-fashioned, but I need to trust you before we have sex."
- "Of course I like sex! And I want to have sex with you! But we can wait."

Safer Sex

- "Before we have sex, I hope we can discuss safer sex practices."
- "Can we discuss HIV status?"

- "I'm going to bring some condoms the next time we meet."
- "When's the last time you've been tested? I was tested last month."
- "I want to tell you that I'm HIV positive. I just want to get it out of the way before we go any further."
- "I can help you put the condom on."

Dating HIV+ and HIV− Men

Basic principle of dating: all men must share their HIV status with their dates before having sex—including telling them the last time they were tested. If a man has never been tested, he must say so. If a man has never been tested but wants and intends to be, he needs to tell his date when, and share the results when they're available. If a man has never been tested and has no desire to be, he must tell this to the man he is dating. Never, ever lie about your HIV status or be vague about it ("Oh, I think I was tested last year"). Share the facts!

Some men will share their sexual histories with one another: "I'm a bottom, but have always used a condom." "I've sucked dick with(out) a condom." "I've had multiple partners, but have always been safe." "I went through a real slut stage, but I'm still HIV negative." "I only kiss and jerk off with guys."

Remember: we all have selective memories, so sexual histories may not be as accurate as we would like to believe. A few men may deliberately tell lies to get you into bed; knowing this should not make you paranoid, but instead give you a heavy dose of reality and inspire you to use your head as you make your way through the world of HIV and safer sex.

Most HIV+ men I have spoken to prefer to date other HIV+ men. In fact, there are now socials and dances exclusively for Poz men. It's not that Pozes don't like Negs, but more often that they've been burned with rejection by them, or prefer the company of men who more directly understand their situation.

One psychotherapist told me that, over the last fifteen years in his practice, he found that 90 percent of Negative guys will reject Poz men after disclosure. Many Negs will never come out and say they rejected the Pozes after disclosure, but the secrets of the therapist's office tell a different story.

Do Negs have a right not to date Pozes? Of course they do. So it's best to be up front on what we want and need in our relationships.

What can a Neg say to a Poz after disclosure?

- "It doesn't mean anything to me. I like you and I'm sure we can do things safely."
- "I prefer not to date Poz guys."
- "I didn't think you were Poz. I need some time to digest this." (But mean it! If you don't mean it, use the bullet point above.)

What does a Poz say to a Neg?

Some Poz guys like to be up front right away in an ad or profile, disclosing their HIV status. Other guys like to meet men in person before disclosing. On what date do we disclose? I recommend disclosure on the second or third date—no later—though some Pozes like to tell men on the first date and get it out of the way. (The one big drawback to disclosing status on the first date is that the whole date can become mired in HIV talk, preventing you from getting the chance to see any other aspect of your date.)

Suggested "Coming Out" Phrases

- "Before we go any further, I need to tell you that I'm HIV positive."
- "This is not easy for me to say, but I have HIV, and I wanted to tell you sooner rather than later."
- "I really like you, so it would be terribly unfair not to tell you that I'm HIV positive."
- "Can we discuss HIV status? Do you want to go first or shall I?"

Cases

Gilbert is HIV+ and never likes to tell men he has the virus. "I can't get rejected. I know if I tell them my status I'll never see them again. I'm sorry I don't tell them, but I can't do anything else. If they ask me, I tell them I haven't been tested."

Gilbert is not alone in not wanting to be rejected. Rejection, particularly when we're lonely and want to experience love in our life, is a terrible feeling. So, though we can't force someone to disclose his HIV status, we can always use safer sex practices, and leave the door open for disclosure in the future.

Henry is HIV– and wants to remain that way. He always asks men their status during their first telephone conversation, e-mail exchanges, or one on one. He doesn't want to date an HIV+ man or someone who's been "promiscuous," to use his word. He also won't go out with anyone who has not been tested. "I'm terrified of AIDS, because I've seen what it's done to people over the years. I won't tongue-kiss guys, and I don't have oral or anal sex, but I can still get off—touching and grabbing and jerking off."

Henry seems to have figured out safer sex practices that work for him, which is key. Some men might take issue with his avoidance of kissing, which is generally thought not to be a means of HIV transmission. Henry must keep in mind, though, that because a person says he's been tested and is HIV−, that doesn't make it true, since the gentleman in question could have contracted the virus *after* being tested, and/or even if he tested negative, there is an incubation period after sexual contact during which the virus might not be detectable. I recommend that Henry join an HIV− support group, where he can talk about his concerns and fears about HIV. (For a candid discussion of safer sex practices, see pages 201–2.)

An interview with a young African American college graduate with HIV

When did you find out you were Poz, and what was your reaction?

I found out I was HIV positive when I was twenty-four and thought I'd be dead in five years. I thought I was damaged goods. I thought my family and friends would leave me, so I joined HIV-positive support groups to understand the psychology of the disease. I started to hang around people who fought the disease and stuck to their drug regimen. My philosophy was that the disease of HIV was about not taking care of yourself.

Do you date Poz and/or Neg men?

I've dated some Neg men in the past, but now I date mostly Poz men—though I'm not closed to meeting Neg guys. HIV is a major issue for most Neg men. I can sense a shift of energy when I disclose my status. They're thinking, "This guy across from me is going to die," and I want to say, "And you're not going to die someday?" Some Neg men who have lost lovers through AIDS don't want to go through the ordeal again. I only date Poz men who don't show any signs of the disease, no one who looks visibly ravaged.

When do you tell Neg guys you're Poz?

It varies. If the first date is short—just some coffee—I usually won't say anything. If I really like a guy, I definitely wait for the second date. Sometimes I will tell people on the first date, depending on my mood and frame of mind. The longest I wait is the third date, and that's rare.

How do you tell them you're Poz?

"I'm HIV positive"—I list it along with my other bio stuff. I don't get all apologetic and weepy. Sometimes I will take my pills in front of them and say, "These are my meds, I'm HIV positive."

Where do you meet guys?

I used to meet guys online. When I didn't reveal my status, I got a lot of trivial responses; it was mostly fun and games. When I put my HIV-positive status in my profile, I got a lot fewer responses, but they were higher quality, and I dated a few guys from that group. Now I only meet guys through other friends and going to events at the gay center.

What is sex like for a Poz man?

Before I have sex with guys, they know I'm Poz. We use condoms for anal sex, and I don't swallow their cum or let anyone else swallow mine. I will suggest they use a condom for oral sex on me; but, if they don't want to, I don't push it. I suck dick without a condom. I can't suck a dick with a condom on—if a guy insists on a condom, I pass on oral sex. I deep-kiss without any worry, as do all the men I've dated. One Neg man I dated wanted to clean himself off immediately after I came on his stomach—it was like radioactive waste for him. When this happens, I try not to have any visible reaction; but, deep down, I feel shame. I know he's scared, but it's hard not to feel hurt.

Dating and Safer-Sex Practices

*Interview with Martin Algaze, director of communication at
Gay Men's Health Crisis in New York City, about safer sex practices*

*Single, dating men want to know what they can do
and what they can't do sexually in the dating scene.*
First of all, there is no such thing as 100 percent safe sex. Oral sex is low-risk, whether you are sucking someone or getting sucked, provided there are no cuts or sores in the mouth. Do not let a man come in your mouth. Kissing is safe. Never have unprotected anal sex. That is the primary way of transmission of HIV for gay men. It takes only one person to infect you.

Why don't some young gay men follow safer sex guidelines?
I believe some young men are definitely letting their guard down and engaging in risky behavior. Younger guys didn't see the first generation of AIDS—they didn't witness the devastating disease. They can't identify with the men who got sick in the eighties and nineties. They think, "If I get infected, I can take medication." But drugs are not a cure, and there is no evidence there's a cure coming soon. Young male models in AIDS prescription-drug advertising glamorize the cocktail regimen, but the drugs are toxic to the body and expensive. And you need to take prescriptions for the rest of your life. Drugs are a stopgap measure.

How do recreational drugs affect HIV awareness?

I notice a big increase in the use of crystal meth in the gay community. I hear that men feel this rush of euphoria—power—and get an insatiable appetite for sex. These powerful drugs alter a man's judgment. Many men don't even remember who they had sex with. These drugs are powerfully addictive: you just can't take them occasionally; you get hooked on them.

Should men get tested?

Yes. HIV is not a death sentence anymore. You have choices on what to do to stay alive. Many men are living with HIV. According to a recent CDC [Centers for Disease Control] report, more than 300,000 people in the United States are infected with HIV and don't know it. They may be having unprotected anal sex.

How has HIV impacted the African American community?

Some African American men don't identify themselves as gay, but do have sex with men. Their sex life is a secret. They may meet guys for sex, or pay for a prostitute, have unsafe sex, and then go back to their girlfriends and wives, and possibly infect them. It is important for these men to find out about their status.

Final Words

I have lost some wonderful and loving friends through AIDS over the years. Not a day goes by that I don't think of them. As a gay single man, you must develop your own set of informed safer-sex guidelines with which you are comfortable. I encourage you to take great pleasure in sex, but to do so safely. We don't want to lose you. We want you to live a happy, healthy, and very long life.

DATING AND ABANDONMENT ISSUES

Abandonment has many faces. Earlier in this chapter, we saw how easy it is to abandon *ourselves* through the Perfect Body Syndrome. Relationships are fertile ground for abandonment issues, since they force us to confront intimacy with other gay men, perhaps for the first time—and the impulse to abandon a relationship at the first sign of trouble may be strong. There are both physical abandonment—in which one gets up and, literally, leaves—and emotional abandonment—in which a man closes off his heart.

Gabriel, a thirty-seven-year-old photographer who grew up in Kentucky, told me that his boyfriend could do anything to him but abandon him. And that's exactly what happened. His boyfriend drank heavily and took drugs, and Gabriel put up with it. His boyfriend would blatantly cheat on him, and Gabriel would look the other way. His boyfriend would verbally abuse him, and Gabriel would accept this, because "He's in pain and I know he doesn't mean it." Why did Gabriel put up with this abuse? "I love him and I know he's had a terrible childhood, and he makes up to me. When he's sweet, he's the best, and when he's nasty, he's the worst. I was taught very early, you've got to take the good with the bad. I know he needs me, and I like the security of a home. I hate being single. To me, it's a fate worse than death. I know my boyfriend has problems. Who doesn't? I know he loves me. He tells me all the time. The sex is great, and he's funny when he wants to be. Deep down, he's a little pussycat."

Gabriel is terrified of abandonment and has an incredible capacity for pain. He will sacrifice anything in order to keep the "stability" of a relationship. This man is not alone, in the straight or gay communities. What people will put up with in order not to lose the security of a mate is mind-boggling. Some men will give up a healthy sex life due to an indifferent mate who has lost his sexual drive. One man told me that his partner would not even allow him to touch him. Another confessed how his partner is cold and distant: "I am more lonely in this relationship than I ever was single. It kills me to be with this cold man, but I can't leave." Another man told me how his partner berates him all the time: "You're an idiot." "You don't know anything about computers." "You're getting fat and ugly." "Don't touch my stuff again."

These unhappy men have lost their sense of self and their dignity. They keep thinking things will get better, but they never do. Why? Because the abusive person needs long-term professional help and, most times, sadly, never gets it.

Johann is thirty-five, and his boyfriend Alfred is twenty-three. Things were blissful for the first four months of the relationship, until Johann found out, through a friend, that Alfred was cheating on him. He confronted Alfred, who denied it and accused Johann's friend of maliciously spreading rumors. Things were never the same. They had less sex and the relationship went into a tailspin. Alfred told Johann that he wanted to leave, but Johann would have none of it. He wanted to work things out. Besides, he couldn't imagine life without Alfred, who was the cutest thing on earth to him and had the charm of ten Matt Damons. Alfred finally confessed that he had met someone else and wanted to separate for a while, at least, but Johann objected. "I don't want you to leave. I'm begging you to stay. I can't live without you. Can't you understand that?" Alfred didn't know what to do. He continued to see his new boyfriend, but lived with Johann, who thought Alfred was going through a "stage"—that he was afraid of real commitment, but that time would bring him around.

One day, Johann found Alfred and his friend having sex in Alfred and Johann's bedroom. The bedroom reeked of pot. Johann told the visitor to leave, and Alfred apologized for the incident. Johann forbade Alfred from inviting his friend to their house again.

Johann put up with an incredible amount of inappropriate behavior in order to keep Alfred, who had become no more, really, than a boarder in a hotel. Johann put it this way: "I love Alfred, warts and all. He's everything I wanted to be and never was at twenty-three. I think he'll come around, once he gets over his infatuation with the nineteen-year-old."

Johann was living with major denial—denial that Alfred would leave him.

Suggestions for Dealing with Abandonment Issues

- Take a "time-out" when things seem out of control. You may wish to spend a night or a weekend with friends in order to cool down and get a fresh perspective on the relationship.
- Establish clear boundaries at the beginning of the relationship. You and your boyfriend may wish to draw up a list of healthy boundaries (e.g., no verbal abuse, no going to bed angry, no use of the telephone during your dialogue, no storming out of the house, alone time guaranteed).
- Establish consequences for any boundary bashing. One man told me he promised his partner fifty dollars if he ever called

him a name—and he never had to pay his partner the money! Another man told his partner, "If you ever physically assault me again, I will leave the house for good"—and his partner never laid a finger on him. I am not saying this will work 100 percent of the time, but it will certainly be good for your sense of self-esteem if you set boundaries.

- Say to yourself, "No one can abandon me without my permission."

- Get to really know men on your dates before you settle down with someone. If you're a man who likes to rush into relationships, give yourself more time.

- Notice the smaller ways in which you allow yourself to be abandoned in a relationship, and verbalize your feelings with your partner about such things as boyfriends being late, not returning your calls, forgetting your birthday, not expressing gratitude for the gifts that you bring to the dating table, etc. Tell your mate: "I need to have a sense that I'm appreciated."

- Don't let your boyfriend walk all over you. Compromise is an important part of dating, but if you have a tendency to give in too quickly, hold the line. Healthy compromise happens when each partner sees the importance and value of the process, and neither partner is "out to win" or to humiliate the other. Swallowing your pride and seeing the other person's point of view with detachment is key to making compromise work. Successful compromise occurs when two caring and committed people sacrifice individual agendas for the sake of growth in the relationship.

CHAPTER 7

COMMUNICATION STRATEGIES
FOR COUPLES

The closer you are to someone, and the longer you have been close, the more you have to lose when you open your mouth.

—DEBORAH TANNEN, *THAT'S NOT WHAT I MEANT!*

If what you're saying is right but you're saying it wrong, it's wrong.

—LIONEL, A FRIEND

For good or bad, our parents are our primary teachers of how we communicate with others in the world. Our secondary teachers include grandparents, siblings, aunts, uncles, religious leaders, teachers, and other influential people in early-childhood development. When you have a disagreement with your boyfriend, all of these influences are present in your actions and reactions. (If you had excellent communications-skill training growing up, you may have the impulse to skip this chapter, but I advise you to continue reading, because there is a high probability that your boyfriend or future boyfriend may lack some necessary communications skills.)

There is never, never has been, and never will be a relationship without problems.

In light of this premise, it behooves all relationship-seekers to find appropriate means of communication to work on these problems. How do you respond to an accusation by your boyfriend that you let a virus enter your computer system, which caused the loss of valuable files? What do you say to a partner whom you perceive to be disorganized around the house, while he thinks you're a little obsessive-compulsive?

Problems don't go away by being ignored. I have an acquaintance who, years ago, upon receiving any bill in the mail, would immediately toss it into the wastepaper basket. She thought that if she didn't look at the bill, "the problem" would go away—till, alas, she was in debt for thousands of dollars.

We may think not talking with our partner will make a specific issue/problem go away, but it never goes away. It just waits to pop up in the most unforeseen of circumstances.

John, twenty-one, didn't like it when his boyfriend lent out his CDs to friends, because they never got returned. He didn't say anything because he has a "nice guy" image, and didn't want to ruffle any feathers. Instead of saying, "Paul, I don't want you to loan out my CDs," he kept his feelings bottled up and secretly seethed when a CD he wanted to listen to was gone. But healthy communication is about addressing issues promptly and saying from the start what we need to say. John finally stopped being the "nice guy" and told Paul that he was not to lend out any of his CDs, to anyone.

TOOLS FOR EFFECTIVE COMMUNICATION

Tool #1—Saying "I'm Sorry"

There was a film in the 1970s called *Love Story,* for which the tag line was "Love means never having to say you're sorry." This lie did a lot of damage to the cause of healthy communication. Love means *having* to say you're sorry. When it is said with sincerity and at the appropriate time, it can be very effective, as the following anecdote illustrates.

Lincoln got into a heated argument with his boyfriend Dennis about money (Dennis's penchant for impulse buying and going into debt), and blurted out, "You're just like your mother!" Dennis was furious that Lincoln had pushed one of his hot buttons— his relationship with his mother—and threw the nearest object, a hardcover book, at him. Lincoln ducked and it missed him. Each looked at the other for a moment, not fully realizing what had happened: that they had both regressed—slipped back into past ways of perceiving, feeling, and thinking—and that they had both lost control.

In a split second, their world had become unsafe, because they were talking about money, and money can bring up all sorts of issues: survival, control, jealousy, fear. Lincoln threw the first "punch"—a barbed comment, and Dennis impulsively—out of anger—literally threw the book at him. It took them a couple of minutes to calm down, and then Lincoln said, "I'm sorry. I shouldn't have said that about your mother." There was about a fifteen-second silence, and then Dennis said, "I'm sorry I threw the book. I hate it when you bring up my mother."

Both men apologized for an incident that had gotten out of control. The "I'm sorry"s de-escalated the situation, bringing momentary calm. Once they came to their senses, Dennis and Lincoln were able to engage in a non-finger-pointing discussion of money.

When we are in relationships with real, live human beings, things don't automatically go smoothly, and if we don't have the communication skills to deal with these circumstances, we're headed toward some major acting out. Acting out (such as the silent treatment, bullying, name-calling, threatening to leave) is the antithesis of healthy communication. Admitting you're wrong, sometimes, and saying, "I'm sorry, honey," even if you don't want to say it, is a sign of emotional maturity.

Tool #2—Paying Attention

We live in a fast-paced society, in which it is far too easy to lose focus and take people for granted. Frequently, we lose the ability to pay attention to one another. Take a look at your own relationship: Does your boyfriend seem a little more withdrawn lately? Has your sex life become too routine? Are you sniping at each other more often? Do you become vague about vacation plans? Do you eat together less often? Do you praise your boyfriend less?

David, pursuing his MBA at age forty-one, was having difficulty doing the term papers and required projects. He'd always had difficulty staying on-task; so, midway through the semester, he felt daunted by the mounting pile of work. Things at the university seemed to be getting out of control. His boyfriend, Harrison, had been traveling a lot on business, and was caught up in his own work. David felt ignored, and thought Harrison was not giving him the emotional support he needed. Harrison would blithely say, "How's the student doing?" and David took that as a dig: *You're just a student, having a grand old time with the college crowd, while I'm the main breadwinner.* One day, David asked Harrison if they could talk, and told him, "I need you to pay attention to me." Harrison, flabbergasted, got defensive. "What do you mean? I'm always here for you, honey!" David said, "I don't think you know what's happening to me at the university. I feel like I'm going under, and I've thought about dropping out." Harrison's jaw dropped. "You're kidding!" "No," David said. "I'm not kidding. I get very scared when it comes to school, and start thinking I'm a big failure. I'm working part-time and trying to get good grades. I'm overwhelmed." David broke down and cried.

What David needed was to express what was really happening to him *emotionally* in his life: that he was scared, that he felt like a failure. When someone verbalizes these feelings with someone they love, it can be very cathartic.

Sometimes we think we're paying attention, but it may be halfhearted at best. For some couples, I actually recommend using an egg timer, giving each other fifteen uninterrupted minutes to talk about what's happening.

Simply listen. Simply pay attention. It pays great dividends.

Tool #3—Monitoring Your Testosterone

When you have two men in a relationship, you have double the amount of the male hormone—testosterone. This can provide gay relationships powerful creative energy and excitement, but it can also be the source of power-and-control issues. When a relationship is negatively "testosterone driven," you'll hear expressions like: "I'm right. Period." "This is the way we always do it!" "Either shut up or I'm out of here." "Mine is the best baseball team. Case closed!" "You have no idea how to pick out colors." "Don't tell me how to drive."

You can't—and wouldn't want to—get rid of testosterone, but you can notice when you're letting your hormones rule your responses. Expressions that will help you in your communications when your testosterone is running high include: "I guess I was wrong." "Let me hear your opinion." "Let's try to compromise on this." "I can be a real jerk sometimes."

What do you say to a partner driven by testosterone instead of reason? "Please calm down. I know we can work this out." "I'm offended when you talk to me in that tone of voice." "I don't see it that way. I'm sorry." "Okay, I think we both need a time-out." And if he persists, just say, "Stop talking to me that way. I don't like it"—as gently as possible.

Tool #4—Watch for Internalized Homophobia

When a man was the victim of a gay-bashing in a small city, his partner was very supportive, showing up at the emergency ward at the local hospital, giving a lot of emotional support after the traumatic event, and contacting a local anti-violence project to report the crime. Though he was outraged at the violence perpetrated on his lover, the partner wondered whether his lover hadn't dressed "too gay," which might have triggered the attack. He told this to his lover about two months later, and his lover was beside himself: "I don't dress 'too gay.' I wear nice clothes, which I like. If wearing a nice shirt and pair of jeans is 'too gay,' then I might as well shoot myself. I don't walk like a macho man—does that mean I'm 'too gay'?" The partner was shocked that his lover reacted so strongly to what he thought was a simple observation about appearance and how to carry oneself in public.

This attempt at support backfired. I told the partner, "Your lover did not do anything wrong. He was attacked for one reason: that he was perceived as being gay. You are very angry about what happened to your lover, and in your desire not to have it happen again, you thought you could tell your lover that *he* has to change something in himself. This is called 'blaming the victim,' and it can't stop the sick, violent, homophobic people in the world."

My client began to recognize his own internalized homophobia. I recommended sensitivity training around this issue at the local gay center. Finally, he was able to communicate to his partner that he was deeply sorry for suggesting that being "too gay" might have instigated the gay-bashing attack. His partner accepted the apology.

How Else Does Internalized Homophobia Come Up?

You're afraid of holding hands in public with your boyfriend.

WRONG COMMUNICATION: Guys don't hold hands. That's for straight couples.

EFFECTIVE COMMUNICATION: I get uncomfortable holding hands in public. I need some time. Can we talk about this later?

You're uncomfortable at the Gay Pride parade.

WRONG COMMUNICATION: All these fags drive me crazy!

EFFECTIVE COMMUNICATION: I'm uncomfortable being here. It brings up a lot of my own insecurities.

Your partner wants to put a couples photo on his office desk.

WRONG COMMUNICATION: I don't want my picture on your desk. I'm not out at my job.

EFFECTIVE COMMUNICATION: I love you very much, but could you hold off on the picture for a little while? This is all too new for me.

Tool #5—Avoid Mind-Reading

Mind-reading is when we think we know exactly what's on another person's mind without doing a reality check first; or, when we want to communicate a want/need to someone without verbally saying it, and just *assume* that the other person gets it. Mind-reading is not an effective means of communication, and only leads to a person *not* getting what he wants and needs.

Say your boyfriend's father passes away and he has to travel back to Texas for the funeral. The death of his father and the trip back home are causing him a lot of grief. You may ask him any of a series of questions: "Do you want me to go back home with you?" "Do you need to be held?" "Is there anything I can do for you now?" "Do you need some time by yourself?" "Can I get you anything?" "Do you want to talk?" By doing that, you're telling your boyfriend that you care for him and that you're available. Don't assume anything. Don't just think: "He probably doesn't want to talk." "He probably doesn't want me to go back to Texas." That's mind-reading. Ask him. Get clarity.

Or, say your birthday is coming up and you want a quiet celebration, not like last year's surprise party with fifty people. You need to communicate to your boyfriend exactly what kind of birthday you want. "Honey, I'd like for us to go to a great Chinese restaurant for my birthday, and celebrate it quietly." Your boyfriend may say, "I thought you had a great time last year, and I already told our friends to save the date for your party!" Your boyfriend *thought* he knew what you wanted and didn't check with you—he was reading your mind. You can say, "Thanks, honey, I did have a good time last year, but this year I want to do something else." The simple act of expressing what's on your mind—and not assuming that people can read it—will move communication to a higher level.

Tool #6—How to Argue/Disagree/Fight

If you don't know how to handle conflict or are unwilling to learn how to handle conflict, the relationship is doomed.

Some men don't want to disagree or argue because they fear abandonment. Deep down inside, they feel the relationship is going to fall apart if there is an argument, or that things will get out of control and they'll end up abandoned. Some men literally have to be told, "Honey, when we argue or strongly disagree, that does not mean I'm going to leave you. If anything, when I can legitimately and rationally argue with you, I feel a lot closer to you."

Some psychologists believe that one reason people get married is so that they can argue without the threat of being abandoned. Most of us have never been taught how to argue with someone we love, so as you get to know your boyfriend, you'd better know how each of you handles disagreements.

Bruce, a thirty-five-year-old building contractor, had been in a relationship with his partner, Michael, for two years. Bruce grew up in a family in which everyone expressed their opinions and differences were encouraged. He used to watch his mother and father argue, and it never got out of hand. There were no insults. No one ever went for the jugular. There was healthy disagreement, and neither mother nor father left an argument feeling diminished or shamed; it was always "kiss and make up" afterward. Bruce received good parental role-modeling.

Michael, on the other hand, grew up with a "rageaholic" father who would terrify the family with his outbursts. His father never got physically violent, but his screaming, menacing gestures and rampages through the house, breaking things, caused deep psychic wounds. So, though Bruce welcomed a good, healthy argument, Michael would strongly resist, and was uncomfortable when Bruce would even raise his voice. Michael feared that Bruce would go off into a rage as his own father had done so often. Michael could not see that expressing healthy anger is different from rage.

Rage is what the repressed man or woman does instead of regularly releasing anger safely. Bruce and Michael agreed that they needed couples counseling to help them learn how to argue. They sought out a gay-friendly therapist who was an expert in conflict resolution. The therapist had them role-play, improvising with mock disagreements. It took them a lot of hard work and commitment to get to the point where they could argue fairly on their own. They drew up their own "Discussing Fairly" guidelines. Michael didn't even want to use the word *arguing,* because it scared him. Bruce had no idea how traumatized Michael had been by his family upbringing. As Michael opened up more to Bruce, he found a new confidence that helped him in all aspects of his life, including dealing with authority figures at his job.

Different styles

Jimmy comes from a nice Southern family in which a gentleman did not argue. His boyfriend, Vince, came from an Italian family in which arguing was a sport. Jimmy would go silent when things got a little rough in their relationship, and Vince would want to talk/argue things out. Vince would say, "Come on, Jimmy, what's the matter? If you have something to say to me, say it." Jimmy saw this as threatening.

If there isn't a safe playing field for arguing/disagreeing, there will be a communication meltdown. I suggested to Jimmy and Vince that they start by using "I" statements when they disagreed/argued. For example, Jimmy first must state what he feels: "I feel angry." "I feel ignored." "I feel annoyed." Then Jimmy must say *specifically* what he's angry/annoyed about, why he feels ignored: "I felt angry" or "I was angry" when "you didn't do the dishes last night," "when you were cruising that guy yesterday," "when you forgot my birthday"; or, "I feel ignored" when "you spend Friday nights with your brother," "when you read the newspaper during supper."

I suggested that he not use words like *always* or *never,* or generalize in any other way, because that is unfair and just tends to escalate disagreements. "I feel angry when you *never* do the dishes." "I feel ignored when you *always* go out with your brother on Friday nights." "You *never* do anything right." Jimmy might be right that Vince never does the dishes, but that line of argument will put him in a box; he'll become defensive and not hear one word after the *always* or *never.*

No one wants to be placed in a corner, with no place to move. We need to give each other some wiggle room—to negotiate instead of merely be aggressive. You may say to your partner, "Please use the 'I' statement," as a reminder to him to "fight fair" when you're disagreeing/arguing about something, rather than act on impulse.

Or you may need to remind yourself. You may have the *impulse* to throw a glass at your boyfriend, you may have the *impulse* to call him a fucking bitch, you may have the *impulse* to threaten to leave him, you may have the *impulse* to say he's done nothing with his life; but rational adult people don't act on impulses. Acting on impulse can damage or destroy even a good relationship.

Any time you're tempted to go for the jugular, take a "time-out" and say to your boyfriend, "I feel a little out of control. I'm going outside [or into the other room] for an hour—I'll be back when I'm a little calmer." If it's your boyfriend who's out of control, say in a firm voice, "Time out! We need an hour or so apart to calm down."

I also recommend that men take five deep breaths—deep inhalations followed by strong "letting go" exhalations—allowing any accompanying sounds to issue from your body ("Ahh!" "Ohh!"). Shake your hands. Move your body freely. Let go of any tension constricting you.

A HANDY FEELINGS CHECK-IN LIST

"I feel . . ."

confused	weak
hurt	edgy
superior	sexy
guilty	energized
daring	pleased

inhibited	exhausted
jealous	joyful
out of control	impotent
frightened	sad
humiliated	loving
embarrassed	angry
inadequate	frustrated
apathetic	disgusted
lonely	envious
abandoned	cynical
bad	inspired
generous	irrational
silenced	depressed

Tool #7—Communicating Gratitude

Some of us take for granted the men whom we love. We *assume* they know that we love them.

Assume nothing—and never for a moment stop expressing gratitude for the man in your life. It may just take saying the simplest of things, like "I love the way you cook pasta," "Thanks for driving me to the doctor's," or "You smell great!"

Other ways we can express gratitude

- You know what I really like about you? (Tell him.)
- I'm proud of you! (And tell him why.)
- You mean a lot to me. (Tell him the reasons.)
- I'm a lucky man because . . . (*Tell him.*)

Other key communications expressions
When your boyfriend is extremely upset over something,
you can say:

- Is there something I've said or done that's made you upset? Please tell me.
- You seem upset. Tell me what's happening to you.
- I'm here for you.
- I support you one hundred percent.
- I can't read your mind. Tell me why you're upset.
- You look tired. Is there anything you need?

When you're not feeling well and are becoming irritable,
you can say:

- I'm exhausted. I need some rest.
- I need a vacation.
- I'm feeling like I need your support right now.
- I need your help.
- I need some time by myself.

Four most frequent questions on communication

1. *How do I tell my boyfriend I want to take things more slowly?* First of all, tell him! Say what's on your mind and what you're feeling *in person,* not by telephone or e-mail: "I'm getting a little scared about how close we're getting." "This is my first real relationship and I want to take it slowly." "You asked about moving in together—I'm not ready for that yet." "It takes me a while to really get to know someone." And let him respond to you. His response, it is reasonable to hope, will be the beginning of your communication as a couple.

2. *How do I tell my boyfriend I want to deepen the relationship?*

First, you need to formulate in your own mind and heart how you want to have a more soulful connection. Do you envision living with this man for the rest of your life? Do you want to raise children or buy a house together? Each relationship has its own movement and pace, and each person within a relationship has his own rhythm. You're not always going to be in sync, but it's extremely important at least to verbalize what you want and need from your mate, and for him to do likewise.

Do you and your mate believe in long-term commitments? Are you on the same page when it comes to financial matters? Do you think couples counseling would enhance the emotional life of your relationship?

Here is what some men have told me they have done to deepen their relationships:

- live together
- share expenses
- start individual therapy
- do couples counseling
- vacation for a month together
- buy a house
- adopt a child
- keep romance alive (e.g., buy each other surprise gifts, massage each other for a half hour without stopping, take showers together)!

A relationship either grows or withers—it never stays neutral. Healthy, satisfying relationships require an enormous amount of work and attention.

3. *Can I date outside the relationship?* When someone is in a relationship, I don't generally advise dating other people. However, it's okay to date several men at once, if things haven't deepened with any one of them.

If you're unhappy with the person you're dating, tell him, so you can deal with the issue(s) at hand. If the problem or problems cannot be worked out to your mutual satisfaction, it may be time to move on. Avoid becoming sneaky: don't date other people behind his back, using your relationship as an emotional security blanket.

If you want to have sex outside your relationship, that is another matter. This has to be talked about. The boundaries must be very clear: "I will meet guys only for brief sexual encounters"; "I will always practice safer sex"; "I will never bring a man home" (if you're living together). I can never recommend sex outside a relationship unless there's total agreement between parties.

4. *I want to end the relationship. How do I do it?* Ending a relationship is never easy. Someone always gets hurt. You must tell your partner very gently, particularly if he has no idea this is coming. Even if you're not living together, always tell the man in person—never by e-mail, and almost never by phone. (Ending a relationship by answering machine, unless there was some violence done to you, is unforgivable. If you feel you must break it off by phone, it's also important to say, "I want to meet with you and talk, for some closure," and follow through.)

Ways to say it

- "This is very hard for me to say, but our relationship is not working."
- "Being together is not working for me. I'm really sorry."
- "You're a great guy and I can't lie to you. I want to date other guys."
- "I'm really confused about where I am in my life and, to tell you the truth, I'm not ready for a relationship."
- "You're a fantastic person. I admire you greatly, but I'm not happy in this relationship. It's nothing you did wrong. I just don't think we're a match."
- "It's hard telling you this, but I want to start dating other guys. You're one of the nicest people I know, but this relationship is not working for me."
- "I'm really sorry this didn't work out, but I need to spend some time by myself."

The way you tell a man you are ending the relationship is crucial to an amicable breakup. Some men may be a little shocked and may need time to process their feelings. Allow that time—it is the most decent and loving thing to do.

What if you're breaking up with a guy because he was a big jerk? You don't have to take his inventory and list all his misdemeanors. When men ask, "What did I do wrong?" they really don't want to know, and you have no obligation to tell them.

If they're in a state of shock, they want comforting more than anything else. Don't bullshit them ("Maybe we can date in the future") or promise them something you can't deliver on ("If you want, we can still go to Palm Springs in February").

And—please—don't have sex. Just a hug.

How to Compromise

Working things out as a couple,
and allowing for and celebrating differences

Simple fact: if, as a couple, you really like each other, you must learn to compromise.

We need to be very aware that, when we move into a relationship, we can't get everything our way. We may like our men a great deal, but they may have idiosyncrasies that drive us crazy. And remember: we each have our own "peculiarities" which may be driving our boyfriends crazy.

I work with couples and the success rate among couples is in direct proportion to the couple's willingness to accept each other's differences. I'm not talking about putting up with a lot of inappropriate behavior, but two healthy men looking into each other's eyes and wanting to work things out.

When there is little or no compromise in a relationship, one or the other of the partners may start to exhibit the following symptoms:

1. pouting
2. mini–temper tantrums
3. passive-aggressive behavior—the silent treatment, withholding love (thinking he has a great shirt on, for instance, but not telling him), smiling and saying that everything is okay when it isn't
4. making negative predictions of where the relationship is going
5. gossiping with friends about the mate

EXAMPLES OF SUCCESSFUL COMPROMISING

Tyrone and Kenny—together three months—live separately

PROBLEM: Tyrone likes to sit in the back of a movie theater, near the exit, because he's claustrophobic. Kenny likes to sit up front.

COMPROMISE: Kenny is aware of Tyrone's claustrophobia and, if the theater is crowded, Kenny is more than happy to sit in the back. Sometimes they'll sit three quarters of the way back, if the theater is not crowded.

PROBLEM: Kenny drives too slowly and cautiously, which drives Tyrone crazy when he's in the passenger seat.

COMPROMISE: Tyrone is now aware that Kenny gets nervous when he has to drive too fast, so doesn't get on his back about it. In fact, Tyrone is open to Kenny taking the more scenic side roads, at times, instead of the superhighways. When they have to get to a place in a hurry, Kenny is more than happy to have Tyrone do the driving.

Pete and Bruce—dating six months— live separately—want to move in together

PROBLEM: Pete's mother calls a lot, and it drives Bruce up the wall when Pete talks with her for an hour at a time.

COMPROMISE: Pete and Bruce started to have designated "private time" during the week, during which there would be no incoming or outgoing calls. Pete also set up some time boundaries with his mother, and Bruce agreed not to be overly critical with or about Pete's mother.

Tom and Dario—have been dating ten months—
do not live together, but are talking about it

PROBLEM: Dario believes that Tom watches porn excessively.
(Tom has about fifty videos.) For the first couple of months,
Dario liked watching porn—he got turned on—but now he
believes it's interfering with their lovemaking. Dario didn't
mind dabbling, but Tom seems fixated on the whole porn
scene, which makes Dario feel ignored.

COMPROMISE: Tom agreed to cut back on his porn watching,
and to play porn tapes only occasionally while making love
with Dario. Dario agreed not to preach to Tom about his use
of porn.

Derrick and Jason—have been dating three months—
do not live together

PROBLEM: Derrick and Jason have a lot of things in common,
except watching TV sports. Derrick loves to watch basketball, football, and hockey, and when they spend weekends
together, Derrick will sometimes watch a lot, which Jason
doesn't like. It makes Jason feel like the "jock's girlfriend."

COMPROMISE: Derrick agreed to cut back on some of the
weekend sports viewing, taping games to watch later in the
week. Both agreed to scheduling non-sports time together
over weekends, so that Derrick doesn't spring any surprises,
like, "Oh, there's a game on this afternoon." Jason agreed not
to criticize Derrick's sports enthusiasm.

Mickey and Sam—dating four months

PROBLEM: Mickey and Sam both love the movies. They enjoy seeing some movies together, but not all. Mickey likes foreign films, and Sam hates them. Sam likes teenage movies with gross-out scenes, and Mickey hates *them*.

COMPROMISE: Mickey and Sam decided to go together only to films which they know they'll both enjoy—and not fight over. Each gave the other permission to see a film alone, or to invite a friend, without guilt.

Roberto and Nate—dating nine months—live together

PROBLEM: Roberto's mother was coming for a visit from Costa Rica, and he invited her to stay for a month at their place—without telling Nate. Nate was furious with Roberto for not informing him, and Roberto got upset about Nate's dissing his mother.

COMPROMISE: Nate and Roberto agreed on a two-week visit at their place for Roberto's mother. Roberto's mom was delighted, because this shortened stay gave her an opportunity to visit friends in another city. And Roberto promised Nate that he would consult him about all guests in the future.

Sleep-Over Arrangements

It's amazing, the number of different "sleep-over" arrangements that have existed in the gay dating community. Sleep-overs are for men who have just recently met, men who have dated for a while and have not yet decided whether to get a place together, and men who, for various reasons, have made a decision to maintain separate domiciles.

Variations and compromises

Denzel and Jake—*together two years*

JAKE: We alternate sleeping over at each other's houses on Saturday nights. We spend Saturday morning till Sunday evening together. We talk by phone every day. We both like our freedom, and when we get together it's always weekend quality time.

Brendan and Norman—*dating six months*

NORMAN: I spend one night a week at Brendan's house in the city, and Friday nights he spends with me in the country. The one night in the city doesn't always work out, due to our work schedules, but we are committed to weekends in the country. Brendan suggested we spend an occasional weekend in the city, and that's fine with me.

Sergio and Dick—*dating two months*

SERGIO: There's nothing set down about when we sleep over: one week it was every night; another, just the weekend. I prefer Dick's place, because it's more spacious and has a big-screen TV. Plus, Dick has a dog, which makes my staying over easier for him.

Frank and Rory—*dating a year*

FRANK: We both have tiny apartments and this is a problem, so we're thinking of getting a place together soon. We always spend the weekends together—usually it's half at his place and half at mine. Weekdays are iffy, since Rory is working on a major project and spends a lot of time on his computer.

Raphael and Oscar—dating three weeks

OSCAR: For the past two weeks, we spent almost every night together at Raphael's place. I live outside the city, and it's more convenient for both of us at Raphael's. It's a one-bedroom with a very large living room and eat-in kitchen.

Phillip and Jonathan—dating one year

JONATHAN: I live with my mother, who is not well. Phillip and I usually spend every other weekend at his place, and it works out fine. We talk and see each other all the time. He comes over a lot for supper, and my mother adores him. We're working on a living situation for my mother, because I want to spend my life with Phillip.

FIVE STAGES OF COMMITMENT

I'm dating different guys. In fact, I love dating, but I never know where I am in the relationship. When is the word *boyfriend* used? When do we cross from dating to being in a relationship? When do I bring him home to my family? When are we committed to each other forever?

—HAROLD, AGE 32

Maintaining healthy communication requires that you verbalize with your mate where it is you stand when it comes to your relationship. In the past, most gay men had no model for building a healthy relationship or acknowledging its stages.

Recognizing and negotiating stages of commitment is essential for any dating man. Many gay men don't know how to approach getting clarity about commitment. The following five stages will help you identify the levels of emotional commitment within your relationship, and will assist you in communicating your needs.

Stage One (1–3 Months): "I Can't Get Enough of Him"
- "We're in heaven."
- "He does nothing wrong."
- status to the outside world: "We're dating."

Stage One is what Hollywood movies are about. It's about sizzle and having fun. Without Stage One, there would be no relationships. I suppose it's nature's way of luring us into a partnership. Stage One is falling in love. It's when our dream comes true. You fall for a man and that's it. You're smitten, and there is this intensity which is overwhelming. It is one of the highest highs in life—or lowest lows, if things don't work out.

Enjoy it as much as you can. Go dancing together. Sneak away for a weekend in Provincetown. Go hiking and make love in the outdoors. Be silly and wacky with each other.

Gifford and Gene
Gifford, a forty-one-year-old producer, came to see me to help him come out of the closet and meet men. He had been in a long-term relationship with a straight, married man for twelve years. They had met twice a month for sex and become very close friends over the years. Gifford kept waiting for his lover to leave his wife, as he had promised, but, over time, Gifford had come to realize this would never happen. "Why would he leave

his wife, when he had the best of two worlds?" Gifford said angrily.

Emotionally, Gifford was like a teenager in the dating and romance arena. I cringed when he told me that he was looking for a knight in shining armor. But he did meet a man who met a lot of his needs. His name was Gene, and they met online. Gifford went on three dates with Gene and thought he was in love. He told me Gene had been looking for a boyfriend for a couple of years.

"Jim, I never met a guy in my life like this one. He's the greatest guy in the world. Real cute, with a great smile. I can't stop thinking about him. He's the guy I'm going to settle down with."

Gifford was going through the "He's fabulous!" stage. I was delighted he was dating and getting to know someone who was gay and single. I told Gifford to take it easy, to enjoy the relationship one day at a time. There was no need to rush.

Pitfalls

Since there is such a magnetic pull in the first three months of being with someone, the urge in most men is to keep the feeling going at all costs. This is impossible. No one can be perpetually "high" with another person; it will only exhaust both of you.

When the rush is gone, some gay singles bolt such a relationship and run to another man, hoping to replicate the first-three-month high. Some men feel that if things are not always at that high peak, there's something wrong with the connection.

Some guys can't resist saying to a partner, "I love you," in Stage One, expecting the other man to say it, too—and when he doesn't, feels rejected. Saying "I love you" *too much* to a date (and potential mate) in the first three months may cost some men the relationship. It has to be said very sparingly, if at all. You can hold another man hostage by loving him to death.

How many times can you say "I love you" before it becomes meaningless? Saying it so much does not mean you're an emotionally mature man—it may mean just the opposite.

So what can you say in place of "I love you"?

- "You mean a lot to me."
- "I really like being with you" or "I love being with you."
- "I've never been happier than being with you."
- "When I'm with you, I'm the most relaxed I've ever been."

Stage Two (3–6 Months): "Getting to Know You"
- testing period
- idiosyncrasies—finding likes and dislikes
- starting to see some warts
- may see red flags
- reconnaissance—gathering information
- one partner gets closer—the other pulls back—then vice versa
- status to the outside world: "boyfriends"

Gifford and Gene
Gifford continued to be very much in love with Gene over the next several months, though their all-night sexual encounters happened with less frequency. In Stage Two, Gene and Gifford were getting to know each other. They shared a love for tennis, which prompted them to join a local tennis group. During Au-

gust, they decided to take a three-night trip to the mountains and camp under the stars (which Gene had loved to do as a kid). Though Gifford enjoyed the first night outside, he asked Gene if they could stay in a cabin the other two nights, and Gene said okay. (Stage Two is also about compromise.)

Soon, though, a couple of chinks in the armor of knight Gene began to appear to Gifford. Gene told him that he was going to South Beach for a week, to see an ex-boyfriend. Gifford got jealous and suspicious.

"Why didn't he invite me? Even if I couldn't get off from work, I would have liked to have turned down the invite. Why a *week* with his ex in the same house? I'll bet they have sex!" Gifford fumed.

I told Gifford to take a deep breath and calm down. I said, "Gifford, you're getting to know someone—how he operates in the world. Gene is visiting his ex in Florida. Did you ask him about his ex?"

"He told me about him. They had an amicable breakup after four years, and he considers him a best friend," said Gifford.

"Okay. They are close friends and Gene wants to visit him. Nothing in that seems to be a red flag. Remember: you're getting to know each other. You don't own him. He's not property. So here's what I want you to tell Gene: 'When you told me you were planning to visit your ex, I got a little jealous, and I'm going to miss you a lot.' That's all. Then let him respond."

Gifford told Gene what he was feeling, and Gene was very touched by his honesty. Gene said he needed some time away from the city, and he hadn't seen his ex in over a year, and, no—

he absolutely had no intention of getting back together with him, nor even the slightest desire to. Then Gene promised to call Gifford each night he was away.

When we fall in love with someone, we are very vulnerable. Even the slightest misstep in word or action can be blown out of proportion. That is why it is important for some men who are new to dating to seek out a competent gay or gay-friendly professional to guide them.

Pitfalls

Stage Two is when the drama queen in either man can emerge. Of the five stages, I believe this to be the most important. It is so easy to give up at this stage! The bloom is off the rose. The slightest difference can be magnified to seem like the beginning of the end of the relationship. And it need not be anywhere near the end at all.

You're experiencing growing pains. Patience is the key virtue for this stage. You need to be careful not to overreact at the slightest change in the other person's behavior. Say to yourself, "Am I willing to accept this man for who he is [reality] or am I only interested in who I imagine him to be [fantasy]?"

Stage Two is the point at which you may notice red flags that help you evaluate whether this man is for you or not: Does he return phone calls promptly? Is he "present" to you during sex? Is there a disconnect that doesn't feel right to you? Does he start to criticize you too much?

Stage Three (6–12 Months): "To Be or Not to Be . . . with Him"

- questioning period
- assessment
- deeper intimacy
- self-sabotage possible
- talk about living arrangements
- status to the outside world: "boyfriends"

Gifford and Gene

Gifford wanted to live with Gene, but Gene said he wasn't ready. For the present, they saw each other two or three times during the week and spent alternate weekends at each other's homes.

Gifford gave Gene a surprise birthday party, and invited friends of both of them. After the guests left, they talked into the early morning hours, sharing things about themselves never before revealed.

Gifford and Gene did everything in bed except have anal sex. There were some awkward attempts at this by Gifford, but his erection would disappear after a couple of minutes. One night, Gene asked Gifford directly to fuck him, and Gifford started to insert his penis, but lost his erection. Both men were frustrated—particularly Gifford, since he felt he was doing all the work.

"I'm real hard, and we're kissing and really getting into it, and I can see Gene wants to get fucked, and I begin putting the condom on and it seems to take an hour, and my dick loses its erection and then I'm thinking, 'Jeez, he thinks I can't keep it up,' and then I give up. We end by jerking each other off."

Gifford told me Gene e-mailed him the next day at work and

said he had enjoyed the previous night but was looking forward to the "fuck of his life" the following weekend. Suddenly Gifford felt pressured.

"What do I do? I don't want to use Viagra. I want to do this myself!"

On that Friday night, things didn't go well. They made love, but there was something missing.

Gifford and Gene were experiencing a Stage Three challenge. They needed to speak about their lovemaking in an honest and trusting way, because Stage Three is all about developing a deeper intimacy. It is about bonding.

Sex is only 10 percent of a partnership, but it affects the other 90 percent. I asked Gifford what he needed from Gene during their lovemaking.

"I want him to want me. I want him to look into my eyes and say, 'Fuck me,' and say it as much as he can. I feel like he expects me to do all the work. I need him to talk dirty to me!"

I asked Gifford at what point he lost his erection.

"It's putting the fucking condom on! I'm putting it on, and I sense Gene is there, waiting."

So I suggested that, next time, Gifford take the condom out of the wrapper right before sex, put it within easy reach, and tell Gene to talk dirty to him. I encouraged Gifford to ask Gene what he might want and need during their lovemaking as well.

In discussing their lovemaking habits, Gene revealed that he considered anal sex to be the "icing on the cake"; that he was also satisfied if Gifford used his fingers, instead. This took enormous pressure off Gifford to perform.

By means of clear communication, their lovemaking improved considerably.

Pitfalls

In Stage Three, partners must be vigilant that the relationship is not being taken for granted. You must ask yourself three questions:

1. *Are you being attentive to each other?* You're no longer living a single lifestyle—there are two human beings who need each other's daily support and respect. For instance, if your partner is having some minor surgery, make sure you ask if he needs you to be there for him or to pick him up afterward.

2. *Do you continue to be affectionate with each other?* Though the intensity of Stage One might have passed, it is imperative that the daily displays of affection not be lost—like saying good-bye to each other with a kiss before leaving for work.

3. *Do you spend some quiet time together every day?* No cell phones. No television. No reading the newspapers. This quiet time may be ordering in and sharing Chinese food for supper. Do not use distractions such as television as a way of avoiding quiet time.

Stage Three is when most couples grow or wither as partners. Unconscious forces beyond your control will make sneak attacks on the relationship, and if you're not vigilant, self-sabotage will rule. That is why it's so important to talk freely with your partner about everything—and, if needed, to get some professional help, either individually or as a couple.

Be humble. Relationships are not easy. It takes an enormous amount of time and effort to maintain a healthy relationship.

Stage Four (1–3 Years): "We're a Couple"
- bonding has taken place
- commitment to one person
- taking a vacation together
- deciding whether to live together or not
- status to the outside world: "We're lovers/partners/a couple."

The first three stages are the most difficult to get through if you're developing a conscious relationship. By conscious relationship, I mean two people acknowledging and accepting both the positive and negative in each other, and who are willing to grow with one another through love and understanding.

When you move into Stage Four, usually after a year, your relationship is no longer a fantasy. The man you're with is a real, live human being. Stage Four requires maturity. If you're not ready for the responsibility of a relationship, you can remain in Stages One and Two with different men forever.

In Stage Four, your sex life may change, though this can vary. Some men think there is something wrong when they and their partner are no longer having sex every day. So be assured: there is nothing wrong. Some couples may have sex two or three times a week, others less often. It's the quality that counts, not the quantity. "Hot sex" can evolve into longer, more intimate sex.

Gifford and Gene

Gifford and Gene decided to move in together. They rented a two-bedroom apartment that was close to each of their jobs. (The extra bedroom was for family and friends.) They agreed that they would take the last two weeks of August for vacation, and go to Toronto, Montreal, and Quebec.

Gifford told me that he had never been happier. Having come from a highly dysfunctional family, he had never felt the peace and security of a home. Gene provided a stability which he cherished.

Pitfalls

Stage Four can provide the home that you always yearned for. However, there will be times when you may pine for your happy-go-lucky single days. You may want to hit the club scene on Saturday night. But this time around, I suggest you bring your partner.

Being partnered is not a life sentence, and does not preclude either partner from doing things by themselves. Gabriel, a thirty-one-year-old banker, loves joining his friends, sometimes, at a local bar, for a drink on Saturday night. He usually doesn't stay past nine o'clock. His partner, Sal—not a bar man—fully supports Gabriel's night out with the boys.

Stage Five (3+ Years): "Growing Older Together"
* commitment to be in a partnered relationship
* option—sharing finances
* option—adopting a child

Stage Five is about doing very adult things. You must decide whether a formal ceremony, such as a commitment ceremony, is right for you. Stage Five is what most men dream about: finding someone to share their life with in a committed relationship.

Gifford and Gene

A big decision is whether to have a commitment ceremony. Gifford and Gene did it big. They rented out a hall and had a gay interfaith minister perform the commitment-ceremony rites. They composed their own vows and exchanged rings, and invited more than a hundred friends and members of their families to share their day.

Challenges

Nothing will challenge us more in a relationship than our beliefs about money. Some men get anxious when the topic of bills, budgets, savings, and investments come up and would rather ignore talking about it. It's important for men in Stage Five to get an excellent gay or gay-friendly accountant/financial adviser to help oversee financial matters. I encourage couples to talk about their investments (however small), mortgage payments, and estate planning.

Every couple is different. Some couples have balanced incomes, others unbalanced. One male couple told me that as soon as they adopted a child, they were going to get joint accounts for everything, and I thought that was a wise move. For couples just beginning to live together, I recommend separate accounts for everything, except household expenses. (It should be noted that there are gay couples who keep separate homes and have no joint accounts. It doesn't make them any less a couple—just different.)

OPEN RELATIONSHIPS

When clients ask me whether open relationships work, I say, "For some couples they do, for others not."

Alex, a forty-two-year-old professor of French, and his partner, Eddie, a thirty-nine-year-old acupuncturist, have been together for twelve years. They are deeply committed to each other and are true soul mates, and have an open relationship—with boundaries.

Alex and Eddie swore to monogamy for the first eight years of their union. They were proud of not cheating on each other and thought it brought them levels of intimacy they could never have imagined before their commitment ceremony. In their ninth year together, they took a vacation to Spain. Alex got a massage by a local, twentysomething masseur, which culminated in Alex getting jerked off. He felt tremendous guilt and told Eddie about it on the plane trip back. Eddie was devastated. "How could you do this? I thought we made a vow to be monogamous!" Alex made a major mistake by saying, "It was the first time I ever did this, and I only got jerked off." Eddie hit the ceiling. "That's so typically gay, rationalizing anything for sex! I hate you for this!"

Alex told Eddie that he loved him, and swore never to do it again. But it didn't work. Alex started having anonymous sex with guys, on an average of twice a month—although nothing high-risk, ever. Alex never told Eddie, for fear that Eddie would leave him.

The sex between Alex and Eddie took place on an average of once or twice a month—usually mutual masturbation or oral sex. Eddie seemed to be satisfied with their sex life, but Alex wanted more. "I have high sexual energy and needed to have sex more than Eddie. I'm amazed he can go without it for so long a time."

Alex couldn't take secrets anymore. "I decided to tell Eddie about my sexual flings—that I needed to have occasional sex outside our relationship. Though it would be a devastating blow to me, I was willing to accept the fact that he might leave me, but I could no longer live a lie.

"When I told Eddie I needed to speak to him about something, I swear he knew (though to this day he denies it) what the topic was going to be. I was shocked that he wasn't shocked! I told him that I wanted to live to a ripe old age with him, but that I need to have sex outside the relationship. He told me that he had spoken to his therapist about the incident in Spain, and that probably he was too harsh on me, but he had been afraid that if he had given me a green light on the matter, I would have turned into another 'alley cat.' We laughed. We cried. Eddie said, 'I always knew you would be the first one to run around—you're a sex machine, Alex.' "

Alex and Eddie went to couples-therapy sessions about the open relationship, and set up these boundaries:

Outside Sex
- Never engage in high-risk sex with an outside sex partner.
- Never spend the night with someone.
- Never have a sex partner call home.
- Never talk about the anonymous sex.

Alex and Eddie's Sex Life

- Continue to be present for each other's sexual needs.
- Continue to touch, massage, and hug each other.
- Set aside one "Romance Night" a month—dinner out, and lovemaking.
- Celebrate their commitment anniversary with friends and family.

Alex and Eddie continue to be in a very strong union. Alex continues to have his sexual encounters. And Alex was both startled and delighted when Eddie asked him if he was open to a threesome with one of his sex buddies.

Would Alex and Eddie's arrangement work for *all* gay couples? Absolutely not. Some couples would be aghast at such an arrangement. Others, who are more traditional, may consider it a violation of their commitment promises/vows.

Each couple must decide what works for them. Here are five models that gay couples use:

- committed monogamous relationship with no outside sex
- committed relationship with occasional outside, low-risk sex, including a "don't ask, don't tell" policy
- committed relationship with agreed-upon promises/boundaries, as with Alex and Eddie
- committed relationship with occasional outside sex, only done as a threesome
- open relationship with no boundaries—with two exceptions: neither partner will engage in high-risk sex, nor will they become boyfriends/lovers with another man

ADOPTING AND RAISING CHILDREN

Adopting a child is one of the most important decisions gay couples will ever make. It is a lifetime commitment. Six questions all potential parents must ask themselves are:

1. Do I love children?
2. Am I willing to commit twenty years or more to raising a child and providing emotional and financial security?
3. Is this a joint decision on the part of both men?
4. Do I live in a state that makes it possible or even relatively easy for gay men to adopt?
5. Can I deal with my child's eventual exposure to homophobia?
6. Can I accept the possibility that my child may have difficulty adjusting to gay parents?

If your answer to all six is a definite yes, I would suggest that you begin researching adoption possibilities. If there is a "maybe" to any of the six, I suggest that you reconsider your decision for a while, do some more reading and research (including talking to other gay parents), and perhaps seek out couples counseling to clarify your intentions and motivation for wanting a family.

A thorny issue not discussed much is: What happens to a child after a breakup? Custody, visitation, and child support are issues that need to be addressed. Choosing family life can never be done on a whim or for status: children are not objects to satisfy *our* needs; they need to be nurtured and supported with unconditional love.

Raising a child is one of the most selfless acts of love any human being can perform in his life. I recommend *The Lesbian and Gay Parenting Handbook,* by April Martin, Ph.D., a comprehensive work covering a number of important topics: choosing a surrogate, adoption, legal issues, raising a child, breaking up, growing up with gay parents, etc.

> *Rodney, thirty-five, and Harold, thirty-nine, are a partnered couple with a three-year-old adopted boy. Rodney told me that, on one Saturday morning, he saw Harold and their son Christopher playing with toys on the floor in the family room. "I was watching Harold and Christopher from another room—they couldn't see me—and I felt so proud to be a husband and father, I started weeping. They were tears of joy. I never thought I could have such love in my life, and that made me very grateful."*

I believe some gay partners receive a special calling to raise a child. This in no way means they are *better* than couples without children.

There are myriad ways to give and receive love. No one should be the judge of another person's life choices.

CIVIL UNIONS

Vermont is the first state in the United States to put into law a civil-union statute granting the rights and responsibilities of marriage to committed lesbian and gay couples. I recently spoke with Walter Zeichner, a psychotherapist from Burlington, Vermont, about what protections this new law offers gay and lesbian couples.

How has the passage of the civil-union bill helped gay people?

First of all, there is now legal protection for gay people in committed relationships. Whether it's visiting your lover in the hospital or dealing with inheritance and health-insurance issues, there is now a law to protect us. In the past, if your lover's family was hostile to you, they could prevent you from seeing him in the hospital. We were always regular, contributing members of society, but now there is equal protection under the law which gives gay citizens an opportunity to become more visible. There's less need to "pass." Passing was a form of oppression. So, the law brought some of us out more. Unfortunately, becoming more visible mobilized the right-wing fundamentalist groups—so it's not been a hundred percent pretty. This is a fight that will go on for many years.

Does a civil union help gay men and lesbians stay together?

For gays and lesbians already in an advanced, committed relationship, the civil-union law can have a positive impact. It can be very validating. The law itself does not make people stay together. Fifty percent of straight marriages end in divorce— a piece of paper does not guarantee permanence.

I believe the law will help our young teenagers more than anybody. They are now growing up with a worldview that says gay people can live together in a union sanctioned by the state. There is now public acceptance. They will not grow up with a lot of the damage that many older gays grew up with in the past, which caused many gay men to have a "get it while you can" mentality. Our young people will go through dating and courting rituals that will prepare them for a long-term relationship.

Keep in Mind

As of early 2003, no other state recognizes the Vermont civil-union law. If there is a dissolution of a union (the word *divorce* is not used in the Vermont civil-union law), partners must deal with the issue of property rights. Since many gay couples have unequal incomes, the person with the highest income would have to pay alimony to the person with the lesser income, so that he or she would be able to maintain the standard of living the couple had together in their union.

If a man/woman leaves his/her partner (from a Vermont civil union) for another person, and does not get a dissolution of the union in Vermont, he or she would be committing adultery under Vermont law—their new relationship would not be legal. This applies, also, to couples out of state who have had a civil-union ceremony in Vermont.

For more information about the Vermont civil-union law, contact the website: www.vtfreetomarry.org

RESOURCE GUIDE

There are more than 121 LGBT (Lesbian, Gay, Bisexual, and Transgender) Community Centers in the United States, and the number is growing. For centers nearest to you in the United States, visit the website: www.lgbtcenters.org. From this website, you can also link to international gay centers.

California
L.A. Gay and Lesbian Center
1625 N. Schrader Blvd., Los Angeles, CA 90028
Tel.: (323) 993-7400
E-mail: info@laglc.org
Website: laglc.org

San Francisco LGBT Community Center
Brian Cheu, Executive Director
1800 Market St., San Francisco, CA 94102

Tel.: (415) 865-5555
Website: sfcenter.org

Colorado

Gay, Lesbian & Bisexual Community Services Center of
  Colorado
234 Broadway, Denver, CO 80203
Tel.: (303) 733-7743
E-mail: glbcscc@aol.com
Website: coloradoglbt.org

Georgia

The Atlanta Gay and Lesbian Center
159 Ralph McGill Blvd., Ste. 600, Atlanta, GA 30308
Tel.: (404) 523-7500
E-mail: jpetty@aglc.org
Website: aglc.org

Illinois

Horizons Community Services
961 W. Montana St., Chicago, IL 60614-2408
Tel.: (773) 472-6469
E-mail: Rogerd@horizononline.org
Website: horizononline.org

Minnesota

OutFront Minnesota
310 East 38 St., Rm. 204, Minneapolis, MN 55409
Tel.: (612) 822-0127

E-mail: outfront@outfront.org
Website: outfront.org

New York
The Lesbian & Gay Community Services Center
208 West 13 St., New York, NY 10011
Tel.: (212) 620-7310
E-mail: info@gaycenter.org
Website: gaycenter.org

Texas
John Thomas Gay & Lesbian Community Center
2701 Reagan St., Dallas, TX 75219
Tel.: (214) 528-9254
E-mail: glccdallas@resourcecenterdallas.org
Website: resourcecenterdallas.org

Washington
LGBT Community Center
1122 E. Pike St., PMB 1010, Seattle, WA 98122
Tel.: (206) 323-LGBT
Website: seattlelgbt.org

ORGANIZATIONS

Below is a list of gay organizations from which you can create your own "ripple effect" and expand your social contacts within the LGBT community, whether through volunteering or participating in specific activities.

Frontrunners

Running and walking, competitive and noncompetitive. "Inclusion, participation, and camaraderie" sums up the Frontrunners philosophy.
Website: frontrunner.org

Lambda Legal Defense and Education Fund

National organization involved in litigation, education, and public policy work.
Website: lambdalegal.org

International Gay & Lesbian Travel Association

Committed to growing and enhancing gay-and-lesbian-tourism business through education, promotion, and networking.
Website: iglta.org

National Lesbian and Gay Law Association

Promotes justice in and through the legal profession.
Website: nlgla.org

International Association of Gay Square Dance Clubs

Clubs throughout the United States. High-energy dancing, using the form of Modern Western Square Dancing.
Website: iagsdc.org

GLAAD (Gay & Lesbian Alliance Against Defamation)

Mission is promoting and ensuring fair, accurate, and inclusive representation of gays and lesbians in all media.
Website: glaad.org

PFLAG (Parents, Families and Friends of Lesbians and Gays)
Provides support, education, and advocacy for more than 460 affiliates in the United States.
Website: pflag.org

GALA Choruses
Promotes gay and lesbian choral movement.
Website: galachoruses.org

Human Rights Campaign
Committed to ending discrimination, securing equal rights, and protecting the health and safety of the LGBT community.
Website: hrc.org

National Gay and Lesbian Task Force
Progressive organization working for the civil rights of the LGBT community, with the vision of and commitment to building a powerful political movement.
Website: ngltf.org

National Gay Pilots Association
An organization of gay and lesbian aviators and aviation enthusiasts.
Website: ngpa.org

Lambda Car Club International
Nation's largest gay-and-lesbian auto club. All you need is a passion for automobiles and everything about them.
Website: lambdacarclub.com

Federation of Gay Games

Association for the international, participatory athletic-and-cultural event held every four years.

Website: gaygames.org

Gay Outdoors

Provides fellowship and recreation through outdoor adventure trips.

Website: gayoutdoors.com

International Gay Bowling Organization

A social organization for men and women who wish to bowl and fraternize in a non-bar environment.

Website: igbo.org

International Gay Figure Skating Union

Network with other gay figure skaters in and outside the United States.

Website: igfsu.org

International Gay Rodeo Association

Members in this rough and rugged sport come from all over the United States. IGRA also sponsors an international dance competition.

Website: igra.com

Rainbow Golf Association

Connect with other gay and lesbian golfers throughout the United States. Join tournaments.

Website: gaygolf.com

Delta Lambda Phi National Social Fraternity
Social, service, and recreational activities for gay, bisexual, and progressive college men.
Website: dlp.org

National Youth Advocacy Coalition
Social justice organization that advocates for LGBT youth.
Website: nyacyouth.org

Gay Spirit Camp at Easton Mountain Retreat
A place to refresh your body, heart, mind, and soul in upstate New York. Retreats, workshops, and social gatherings.
Website: gayspiritcamp.com

Single Men's Weekend in Provincetown
A yearly November weekend of fun, education, and romance.
www.singlemensweekend.com

DIRECTORIES, GUIDES, TRAVEL

Gayellow Pages:
www.gayellowpages.com

Damron Guides:
www.damron.com

Odysseus—International Gay Travel Planner:
www.odyusa.com

Out & About Travel Newsletter:
www.outandabout.com

MATCHMAKING SERVICES

Meeting people online does not have to be cold and utilitarian. The websites below will help you to connect with other singles quickly and easily.

Edwina.com
Match.com
Nerve.com
PlanetOut.com
Salon.com
Timeoutny.com

OTHER RESOURCES

If you want a telephone or in-person consultation session with Jim Sullivan, call (212) 946-6560.

Jim is available for workshops/seminars for colleges, faith communities, health organizations, business groups, and special events. E-mail: Jsulli9028@aol.com, or write Jim at London Terrace Station P.O.B. 20157, New York, NY 10113. Visit Jim's website for upcoming events: www.gaydatingcoach.com

BIBLIOGRAPHY

Gay-Specific

Clark, Don. *Loving Someone Gay.* Berkeley: Celestial Arts Publishing, 1997.

Ford, Michael Thomas. *It's Not Mean if It's True.* Los Angeles: Alyson Books, 2002.

Isay, Richard A. *Becoming Gay: The Journey to Self-Acceptance.*
   New York: Pantheon, 1996.

Kaufman, Gershen, and Lev Raphael. *Coming Out of Shame.*
   New York: Doubleday, 1996.

Martin, April. *The Lesbian and Gay Parenting Handbook.* New
   York: HarperCollins, 1993.

Signorile, Michelangelo. *Life Outside.* New York:
   HarperCollins, 1997.

Vera, Veronica. *Miss Vera's Cross-Dress for Success.* New York:
   Villard, 2002.

Wolfe, Daniel. *Men Like Us.* New York: Ballantine Books,
   2000.

Fiction

Baldwin, James. *Giovanni's Room.* New York: Modern Library,
   2001.

Spirituality

Dass, Ram, et al. *Still Here.* New York: Riverhead Books, 2000.

De la Huerta, Christian. *Coming Out Spiritually.* New York:
   Tarcher/Putnam, 1999.

Harvey, Andrew, ed. *The Essential Gay Mystics.* San Francisco:
   HarperSanFrancisco, 1997.

Huber, Cheri. *Be the Person You Want to Find.* Mountainview,
   California: Keep It Simple, 1997.

Levine, Stephen. *A Year to Live.* New York: Bell Tower, 1997.

Moore, Thomas. *Care of the Soul.* New York: HarperCollins,
   1992.

Ruiz, Don Miguel. *The Four Agreements.* San Rafael,
   California: Amber-Allen Publishing, 1997.

Thompson, Mark. *Gay Soul.* New York: HarperCollins, 1994.

Tolle, Eckhart. *The Power of Now.* Novato, California: New World Library, 1999.

Psychological

Beattie, Melody. *Finding Your Way Home.* New York: HarperCollins, 1998.

Hendrix, Harville. *Getting the Love You Want: A Guide for Couples.* New York: Henry Holt & Company, 1988.

Lee, John. *Growing Yourself Back Up.* New York: Three Rivers Press, 2001.

Mellody, Pia. *Facing Codependence.* New York: HarperCollins, 1989.

Tannen, Deborah. *That's Not What I Meant!* New York: Ballantine Books, 1986.

Health

Hay, Louise. *You Can Heal Your Life.* Santa Monica: Hay House, 1984.

Marfuggi, Richard A., M.D. *Plastic Surgery: What You Need to Know.* New York: Penguin Putnam, 1998.

Dating and Romance

Handley, Helen, ed. *The Lover's Quotation Book.* Wainscott, N.Y.: Pushcart, 1986.

12-Step Recovery

Carnes, Patrick. *A Gentle Path Through the Twelve Steps.* Center City, Minnesota: Hazelden, 1993.

Kurtz, Ernest, and Katherine Ketcham. *The Spirituality of Imperfection.* New York: Bantam Books, 1994.

ABOUT THE AUTHOR

JIM SULLIVAN is a national seminar leader and dating and relationship coach with twenty-five years of counseling experience. He holds master's degrees in counseling from New York University and in religious studies from Manhattan College. He lives in New York City and can be reached at www.boyfriend101.com.